P9-DJU-501

Saving Henry

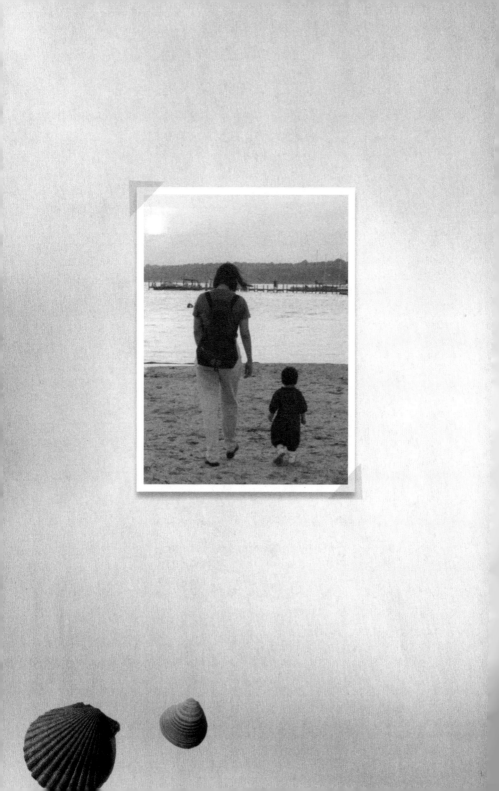

Saving Henry

A Mother's Journey

Laurie Strongin

HYPERION

New York

Copyright © 2010 Laurie Strongin

All photos courtesy The Strongin Goldberg Family

All rights reserved. No part of this book may be used or reproduced in any manner whatsoever without the written permission of the Publisher. Printed in the United States of America. For information address Hyperion, 114 Fifth Avenue, New York, New York 10011.

"Beer Run" Written by Todd Snider & Keith Christopher. Published by Jipco Music o/b/o itself & Elmo Buzz Songs (BMI)/Bug Music o/b/o Bag Daddio Music (BMI).

"Beer Run" Words and Music by Keith Christopher, Julie Ann Doyle, Michael Maye and Todd Snider. © 2002 BAG DADDIO MUSIC (BMI), ELMO BUZZ SONGS (BMI), JEWEL TONES MUSIC (BMI), JIPCO SONGS (BMI) and MUMBA MUSIC (BMI)/ Administrated by BUG. All Rights Reserved. Used by Permission.

Library of Congress Cataloging-in-Publication Data

Strongin, Laurie.
  Saving Henry : a mother's journey / by Laurie Strongin.
    p. cm.
  ISBN 978-1-4013-2356-1
 1. Goldberg, Henry Strongin, 1995–2002. 2. Strongin, Laurie.
3. Strongin, Laurie—Family. 4. Fanconi's anemia—Patients—Biography.
5. Fanconi's anemia—Treatment—Case studies. 6. Mothers and sons—
United States. I. Title.
  RC641.7.F36S77 2009
  369.196'1520092—dc22
  [B]
        2009021551

Hyperion books are available for special promotions and premiums. For details contact the HarperCollins Special Markets Department in the New York office at 212-207-7528, fax 212-207-7222, or email spsales@harpercollins.com.

Design by Susan Walsh

First Edition

10 9 8 7 6 5 4 3 2 1

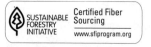

THIS LABEL APPLIES TO TEXT STOCK

To Henry, my hero

Jack and Joe, two magnificent boys who fill
my days with wonder, and my life with joy

And Allen, my partner, my love

Acknowledgments

Saving Henry, the book and the pursuit on which it is based, would not have been possible without the love and encouragement of my devoted husband Allen. I married Allen at a time when I was fortunate enough not to understand true hardship and what it took to confront it. Throughout Henry's life and in his death, the wisdom of my decision to say "yes" to Allen's proposal of marriage was reaffirmed over and over again. Despite the depths of our shared and individual sorrow, and our differing ways of coping with Henry's death, Allen understood and supported my need to tell Henry's story. He read every draft, and over the five years that I worked on this book, there were many. He encouraged me when I needed it; he celebrated my accomplishments like they were his own. For all this and more, I am forever grateful and very much in love.

Jack and Joe, I wrote this book for you. I want you to know how hard Dad and I fought to save Henry's life, not only because he is our son, but because he is your brother. We can never know the pain of losing a big brother so young, but the mere thought of it gave us the strength to keep fighting for Henry's life, even at the most difficult of times. Inside these pages is the story of our family and the backdrop of your unusual childhood. From the moment of each of your births, you have filled my days with joy, pride, and wonder. My love and admiration for each of you knows no bounds. I love you forever.

Mom and Dad, your unconditional love is all I need, and you have given me that and so much more. Thank you for always believing in me and for welcoming Allen and my boys into the family with open arms and open hearts. Ted, thank you for embracing me and taking care of all of us. Phyllis, we miss you terribly.

I know Henry's life and death were a source of incredible pride and sorrow for my sister Abby Cherner, my brother Andrew Strongin, my sister-in-law Jennifer Low, and your spouses Andy Cherner, Tracey Goldman, and Daniel Low. You and your children Michael, Rachel, Joshua, and Noah Cherner; Emma and Sam Strongin; and Hannah Low brought so much joy to Henry and continue to provide comfort to all of us. We are lucky to have you in our lives.

To all of you who fed us, comforted us, traveled miles and miles to hold our hands, canceled and restarted the newspapers, sent us gloves and snow pants, loved us and our kids, you know who you are and I will never forget your kindness. We knew we couldn't save Henry or ourselves alone, and you ensured that we never had to.

In the summer of 2008, Hope for Henry, the foundation Allen and I started to make really sick kids really happy, even for a moment in time, had caught the interest of two men, Preston Padden and Matthew Gerson, both of whom were committed to helping kids like Henry. Over dinner, they asked to know more about the inspiration behind Hope for Henry. So I told them Henry's story. "That would make a good book," Preston said. The next day I sent him the manuscript that eventually became *Saving Henry*. Thank you both for believing in me and for putting my precious work in the hands of Ellen Archer at Hyperion. Within days, *Saving Henry* made its way to Leslie Wells, who embraced its potential and worked tirelessly and devotedly to help me create the book you are holding in your hands. I want to thank Heather Schroder for all you have done to ensure *Saving Henry*'s success; and Aimee Molloy for helping me get to the finish line.

I owe a debt of gratitude to Lisa Belkin, Debbie Blum, Carol Blymire, Jeffrey Goldberg, Chuck Lane, David Martin, and Ben Wittes, all expert writers who saw *Saving Henry*'s potential early and often, encouraged me to keep writing, and believed that one day this book would find a home. It is better because of all of you.

And to the doctors without whom we wouldn't have had a chance. Dr. Arleen Auerbach, Dr. Al Gillio, Dr. Mark Hughes, Dr. Zev Rosenwaks, Dr. Aziza Shad, and Dr. John Wagner, thank you for doing your very best to save Henry. You gave us all hope, even, maybe especially, in the darkest moments.

Finally to Henry. Being your mom has been an extraordinary gift. I continue to marvel at your incredible merry-making and the immense impact of your too-short life. I carry you with me wherever I go.

Contents

Contents

Saving Henry

Henry's Favorite Things

- His girlfriend, Bella
- Catching fireflies
- Collecting shells
- Bathing by candlelight
- Wearing (and eating) candy necklaces
- Fireworks
- M&M's (plain, not peanut)

TRUE LOVE

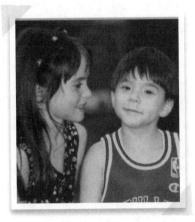

*Henry and Bella share a quiet moment
on a warm summer evening*

*T*he list of Henry's favorite things is lengthy and wide-ranging. Marbles, watches, and *Tom and Jerry* cartoons. Batman, Cal Ripken, and a Pokémon named Charizard. Skittles, chocolate croissants, and garlic bread. Having a lemonade stand, taking a bath by candlelight, and making telephone calls.

But at the top of the list of Henry's favorite things is a little girl who is as beautiful as her name: Bella.

As Henry got sicker and sicker year after year, his list of favorite things grew to include more unusual items: electric blankets, portable urinals, root-beer-flavored anesthesia.

Still, Bella Herold, the love of Henry's life, was always, without question, at the top of his list.

Henry met Bella in September 1998, on one of his first days as a member of the Sunflower class at a preschool in northwest Washington, DC. Bella was the teacher's helper, the teacher being her mother. By the time I arrived to pick him up, Henry was in love. At two and three respectively, Henry and Bella's dates were supervised. And there were lots of them. Sometimes she came over to our house to play soccer, or tag, or to go out for an ice-cream cone. Sometimes he went to her house for pizza or swimming, or to meet her new hamster. Each October, they celebrated their birthdays together. Henry gave her jewelry. Bella gave him Batman T-shirts.

"Mom, come see what we did!" Henry yelled one afternoon from the front porch where he and Bella were shooting stomp rockets into the street and over a neighbor's house. "We wrote our names, and Jack's, too!" To this day, the bricks on our front porch are covered with faded pink, blue, and yellow chalk advertising "Henry," "Jack," and "Bella," alongside hearts, stars, and a few simple math equations.

Henry spent a lot of time with Bella; her mom, Liane; and her sisters. One warm summer day in June of 2000, Bella invited Henry, then age four, to go swimming at the Inverness Recreation Club in her suburban Maryland neighborhood.

"See you later, alligator," I called out to Henry, as my husband, Allen, and I drove away.

"While, while, crocodile," he replied.

According to Bella's mom, Henry and the girls swam and played in the pool for a long time. When they were done, Henry jumped out of the pool and took off his wet bathing suit, leaving him naked, in close proximity to the girls and all the other swimmers and nonswimmers at the pool that afternoon.

"Mom," Bella whispered insistently, "Henry's naked. Get him to put his clothes on, or at least a towel."

Liane offered up both possibilities, to which Henry replied, "It's OK. I'm good."

When it came time to go back home for lunch, Henry walked with Bella and her family from the pool several blocks to their house, completely naked, without a care in the world, an expression of the self-confidence that would serve him well in the years to come.

When I asked Henry what he liked most about Bella, he said, "Everything." From the sweet smile on her freckled face to her long straight brown hair that was often adorned with flower-covered headbands to her slightly shy and down-to-earth personality, she was more than just likable. So much so that Henry stopped saying that he was going to marry me. So much so that I didn't even mind. The only other girl who ever tempted Henry was Snow White, whom he spent a few days chasing around Walt Disney World. But even she, the Fairest of Them All, couldn't compete with Bella.

As Henry got older, and a little bit sicker, Bella—along with new movie releases, trips to the Pokémon Center in New York City, wax bottles from Candy Kitchen in Rehoboth Beach, Orioles games, and birthday parties—was a driving force behind his "Let's Just Do It!" attitude and his unwavering and continuously tested determination to get out of the hospital. When Bella called to invite Henry to her ballet recital in June 2002, nothing was going to stop him from being there.

Henry had recently graduated from kindergarten. Like many six-year-olds, his portfolio of artwork was filled with white paper covered with colorful Magic Marker print that read HENRYHENRY-HENRYHENRYHENRYHENRY. His handwriting was beautiful, earning him a "P" from his teacher, for Proficient. He was great at drawing hearts and flowers, and I have stacks of notes advertising his love for me. My favorite is on a yellow-lined Post-it that has a picture of us and the words HENRY. I LOVE YOU MOMY. I WILL OOWET LOVE YOU. ("Oowet" is Henry for always.) Later, he made a poster publicizing his love for Bella. It's a beautiful picture of them, two stick figures with huge smiling faces, along with three words, all capitalized: *HENRY. BELLA. BELOVE.*

Henry and Bella were well into the fourth year of their courtship, and things were going strong. Henry's bedside table featured a picture of Henry in his number 23 Michael Jordan Chicago Bulls jersey, and Bella in a pretty blue dress with little white flowers. They had spent the afternoon playing soccer together in our backyard. At this moment in time, Henry is kissing Bella's cheek and she is smiling. Although you can't tell by looking at the picture, they are also holding hands. Bella, too, had a picture of the two of them in her room at home. When Bella sent Henry cards, for his birthday or to plead with him to Get Well Soon, she signed them "I ♥ U, Bella"—which was all he needed to know.

Early one warm and sunny morning, I felt Henry's presence by my bed. When I opened my eyes, there he was. Sporting a yellow button-down shirt, blue blazer, and khaki pants, Henry was dressed and ready to go.

"Mom, get up," he was whispering. "We need to go see Bella. We need to go now. And don't forget what we talked about." The night before, Henry explained that we would need to leave a little early because he wanted to buy flowers for Bella to give to her after her dance recital. I looked at the clock: 6:32 a.m. We had three hours, twenty-eight minutes.

Henry picked out the most beautiful white roses he could find, and we arrived at the auditorium in plenty of time. Henry joined Bella's mother, sisters, and grandparents to watch her dance. I had left—it was a date, after all—but Bella's mom, or "Little L," as Henry affectionately called her, summed up Henry's expression as "mesmerized." I'm not sure if she was describing how he appeared during Bella's performance or afterward, when she shared the same seat with him for the remainder of the recital.

On October 25, 2002, Henry's seventh birthday, he and Jack, his younger brother, were treated to a private performance at our home by a magician named Turley. Henry's white blood cells had failed him again, necessitating yet another prolonged period of isolation from friends, school, movie theaters, ice-cream parlors, amusement parks—just about everything and nearly everyone that made life worth living. Turley was able to draw laughter and awe from the boys, but despite being the master of making a triple-scoop ice-cream cone with jimmies from stale milk and ants, Henry knew that a birthday party with no friends isn't much of a party at all.

Later that evening, Henry whispered in my ear, "Mommy, it's my birthday and I really want to see Bella." He added, "Don't tell anyone. Definitely don't tell Dr. Wagner." Henry knew that I would understand that a date with Bella could more than turn the day around. I asked Allen to take Jack upstairs and get him ready for bed. Within minutes, Henry and I were in the car. Destination: Bella's house. I knew that the risks associated with seeing Bella were nothing compared to the rewards. If we snuck in a visit with Bella from time to time, Henry would keep fighting, and one day he would get better.

For hours, Henry and Bella sat on her couch and watched TV, played games, talked, and laughed. I took a few pictures for Henry to add to his collection and to record yet another chapter in the amazing love story of my spirited son and his sweet girlfriend.

Henry's Favorite Things

- Pokémon trading cards, especially those with 90 hit points or more

- Nicknames like Uncle Stinky, Nicky Picky, Ari-bo-bari, and Jackie-boy

- Riding around the neighborhood in his Radio Flyer wagon

- Peter Pan

- Batman Band-Aids

- Sea kayaking with Dad

- Blowing out candles

2

BECOMING HENRY'S MOM

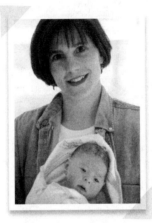

Holding Henry close to my heart

This is a story about the power of love, and the promise and limits of science. It is a story in which politics, ethics, and advances in reproductive genetics collide. It is a story of the group of physicians who took our family to the outer edge of science and into the whirlwind of national controversy. It is a story about a family's search for a miracle, and the children who lived to tell the story. Finally, it is a story of a remarkable little boy who taught me and countless others what is important and what just doesn't matter at all; who showed me how to live well and laugh hard even in the face of odds you'd have to be crazy—or full of hope—to bet on.

It was October 25, 1995, and we were in an operating room at George Washington University Hospital in Washington, DC: Allen and me; our obstetrician, Richard Beckerman; a neonatologist; several medical interns; and delivery-room nurses—a not-so-intimate group of ten or so. My relatively uneventful pregnancy had culminated with a diagnosis of intrauterine growth retardation (IUGR), meaning that my baby had stopped growing. I first learned about IUGR and its potential threat to my baby—mainly, low gestational weight—at my thirty-six-week checkup. For ten days I endured a series of fetal stress tests, all of which were normal. But because the baby was breech in addition to the IUGR, Dr. Beckerman decided to deliver by Cesarean section when I was thirty-seven and a half weeks pregnant. Although I was nervous, any concern about the baby's health was mitigated by normal blood tests and sonograms earlier in the pregnancy and the absence of any pregnancy-related complications.

That morning, numb from the chest down, I lay with a surgical sheet draped over me, preventing me from seeing a thing. Allen stood by my side and we waited for the moment when we could hold our first baby for the very first time. I had planned to give birth naturally, so lying there, unable to feel or see anything, was disconcerting.

"What's going on?" I asked Allen, who kept releasing my hand and drifting away to witness the wondrous moment when he would become a dad. "Is everything OK? Can you see anything? Is it a boy or a girl?" I wanted to be part of the action, which was ironic since at the moment, temporarily at least, I had the starring role.

Even more important, I wanted the information that would allay any lingering concerns I had about the baby's health.

Finally, I heard a sweet little cry.

"It's a boy!" exclaimed Dr. Beckerman. "And he's peeing on me."

At five pounds, Henry Strongin Goldberg was a healthy size, considering the IUGR. I was immediately, and enormously, relieved. I had been worried that if he were only three or four pounds, he might have had to spend a few additional days in the hospital—a concern that, at the time, seemed devastating. As the nurses tended to Henry, the doctor told us that his Apgar scores—a commonly used evaluation of a newborn's physical condition immediately after delivery—were around nine. This was wonderful news, because a baby who scores a seven or higher on the Apgar test is generally considered in good health. But as one of the doctors presented Henry to Allen and me, clean and wrapped in a blanket, I noticed a tiny extra thumb on his right hand. I reached out for him, but the doctor, also having noticed the extra thumb, whisked Henry away to take a more thorough look.

I never even got to hold him.

The waiting room, meanwhile, was filled with our family: Allen's and my parents; my brother, Andrew; my brother-in-law, Andy; and my sister, Abby, who was, at that moment, nine months pregnant with her second child and experiencing early contractions. They sat and waited, watching television, sipping cold coffee, and playfully placing bets on the gender of our baby, all of which my father was recording on video to make certain he had evidence when the time came to pay up. My brother was sure it was a girl, the others said a boy, while Allen's mom, Phyllis, had the good sense to refrain from weighing in. The conversation was interrupted by the arrival of a nurse pushing a newborn baby down the hall in a plastic bassinet.

"Who do we have here?" asked my dad, leaning over to get a closer look at his new grandson. "Have you looked at him yet? I mean, he's got all the right number of appendages in the right places?" he teasingly asked the nurse, just as he had when my sister, brother, and I were born many years earlier.

"He does have an extra thumb," the nurse replied. "But apart from that, everything seems to be in the right place. Better to have more than less, I suppose." Without a pause, the conversation continued: how cute Henry was and who he looked like. No one seemed to realize that with that extra thumb would come a future that none of us had ever imagined.

"He's adorable, look at him!" exclaimed Abby.

"He's got Laurie's nose," added Andy.

Allen arrived, still wearing the scrubs he had donned in the surgical suite. After a round of hugs and handshakes, Allen looked around the room at the faces of his family. "Did you notice his finger?"

"What finger?" my dad asked. Like the others, he hadn't absorbed the nurse's news.

"Well, he's going to throw a mean fastball because he's got six fingers," Allen replied. Again, little reaction. None of us knew what an extra thumb could mean. Instead, everyone was moving to the window outside the nursery, where they crowded together to stare lovingly at Henry, lying in his bassinet in a diaper and a soft blue-and-pink striped hat.

I've watched the video of this scene so many times, I know it by heart. It's here when Henry's pediatrician appears in the hallway and shares the following news: "Henry's having a little bit of a problem with the lungs . . . so we're going to close the curtains now." With that, the video abruptly goes dark.

. . .

While I was wheeled from the delivery room to another room upstairs, several new doctors were with my son, conducting a battery of tests, trying to assess his wellbeing. Allen took turns at each of our bedsides. I had given him a video camera as a "new-dad" gift a few days earlier and, with that in hand, he rushed back and forth, filming and then showing me video of our firstborn son. He had a head of lovely brown hair and perfectly pink skin. And he was strapped to an oxygen mask, encased in a bubble, in intensive care. That's how I first got to know Henry.

That afternoon, with my family around my bedside, close friends stopped by my room to congratulate me and meet the baby. Becca Knox and Erica Antonelli, my friends from high school were there; along with Val Syme, one of my closest college friends. The room was filling with flowers, which Allen kept putting in the bathroom because of his allergies, and the phone kept ringing. As much as I accepted people's good wishes and congratulations, I was increasingly filled with dread. I still hadn't met my son. I couldn't tell anyone what was wrong. I couldn't even answer the question of who he looked like. Finally, a doctor I hadn't met before walked into the room. He introduced himself, and upon hearing his title—Dr. Thomas Hougen, head of cardiology at nearby Children's National Medical Center—and registering the look on his face, Allen asked everyone to wait in the hallway. After closing the door, the doctor explained that Henry had a serious, but correctable, heart defect called tetralogy of Fallot.

Those three words meant nothing to me. As the doctor spoke, repeatedly mentioning Henry's heart, all I could think was that this man had to be in the wrong room, talking to the wrong mom, about the wrong baby. "This doesn't make any sense," I thought to myself. "It's just an extra thumb." It was as if I were an observer of my own life, like an actor in a bad made-for-TV movie. But Dr.

Hougen kept saying the name Henry, and he kept talking as if he were saying something we needed to know. I looked over at Allen, at the concern creasing and folding the features of his face. I reached down and touched my deflated belly, swollen and pulsating with life just hours earlier. I fingered the thick bandages covering the sutures that held my abdomen together. With that, all the benefits of denial vanished.

Dr. Hougen, a softspoken and kind man, gently and carefully explained that our son, barely six hours old, had four different heart problems. The first was ventricular septal defect, which was a hole between the two bottom chambers, or ventricles, of the heart. The second was pulmonary stenosis, or an obstruction at or below the pulmonary valve. Also, the aorta (the major artery from the heart to the body) lay directly over the ventricular septal defect, and the right ventricle was more muscular than normal. I tried to listen carefully as he explained everything, but as someone whose last hospitalization had been on the day she was born, I just could not make sense of what he was talking about. It was like he was an adult in a *Peanuts* cartoon, emitting *"blah blah blah,"* speaking in a language I didn't understand. When Dr. Hougen showed us pictures of a normal heart and a heart with tetralogy, I couldn't even tell the difference.

In short, Henry was what is known as a "blue baby." Because tetralogy of Fallot causes lower than normal levels of oxygen in the blood, it causes babies to turn blue. There was a good chance that Henry could have a "blue" episode in the next couple of days, weeks, or months. If he did, he would need emergency surgery to insert a shunt into his heart, which would provide adequate blood flow to his lungs as a temporary fix. And even if he didn't have an episode, when he reached twelve pounds, he would still need to have the defects fixed through open-heart surgery. I listened, but I don't think I heard anything beyond "Henry" and "open-heart surgery."

My body started shaking uncontrollably. I was desperate to hold this Henry he was talking about; scared that I would never have the opportunity.

"Please," he said with a look of genuine tenderness, "try not to worry. Henry is going to be OK. This is correctable. It has a ninety-nine-percent success rate. And I know the perfect surgeon."

I wanted to trust him, to find some comfort in that number—*99 percent*—but I was too busy fighting the terror escalating in me. As a first-time mother at thirty years old, I felt ill-equipped to care for a healthy baby, let alone one with a serious heart problem and an extra thumb. I didn't even know how to change a diaper. With the help of friends, we had chosen a pediatrician, but we didn't have a referral source for pediatric heart surgeons. Everyone we knew had healthy babies.

Dr. Hougen was barely out the door before Allen was right beside me. "Laurie, he's going to be OK," Allen said as he turned on the video camera to show me, once again, images of Henry taken in the nursery one hour earlier. "Just look at our little guy. He's so beautiful. He isn't going to turn blue. And you heard Dr. Hougen. They can fix his heart. You can't get much better than a ninety-nine-percent success rate. He's going to be OK."

"How do you know?"

"I just do," he said confidently. This was the first test of a soon-to-be-well-honed coping mechanism that was partly male and mostly Allen: an ability to fast-forward past the terrible what-ifs and land squarely on top of the best-case scenario. *He's going to be OK.* As our family and friends streamed slowly back into our room, a look of concern on their faces, I decided that I was going to believe Allen and those five little words. I was going to believe in them with everything I had.

My mom and dad stood at my shoulder, my mom's hand on my hair. I looked up into their loving, worried faces.

"What happened?" my mom asked.

I practiced: "He's going to be OK."

Of course, I'd be lying if I said that my confidence lasted very long. That afternoon, my brain shuffled through everything I did while pregnant, searching for a reason this was happening; for the possibility that this was all somehow *my fault*. I ate well. I took all my vitamins. I got enough, but not too much, exercise. I avoided caffeine, alcohol, and secondhand smoke. I had done everything right. It just didn't make sense. I couldn't lie there anymore, driving myself crazy with these thoughts, missing out on the first hours of my son's life: A boy I'd never met, and whom I now missed so much it hurt. I had been instructed to stay in bed, given the stitches newly placed to hold my abdomen together, but I willed my body to sit up. I called the nurse, who joined Allen in slowly placing me in a wheelchair. A few minutes later, and sixteen hours after Henry was born, I got to hold my boy.

In a darkened room, well past midnight, in the neonatal nursery, Henry wrapped his tiny fingers around mine and latched his lips onto my breast. My milk began to flow through his body, and I felt a love that I never knew existed. It was quiet and peaceful and safe. There were no unfamiliar people, whispering unfamiliar words. Just a new mom, a new dad, and a beautiful newborn baby. I felt Allen's arm around my shoulders and my son's body in my arms; warm, lovely, and safe as I rocked him to sleep.

Two days later, Allen pulled our Isuzu up to the hospital entrance, where I was waiting in a wheelchair holding Henry. Allen tenderly put Henry into his new car seat and helped me into the seat in the back, next to Henry. The sun's warm rays filtered into our car, and the natural light was uplifting. Allen drove below the speed limit, perhaps for the first time in his life, with his left hand on the wheel and his right reaching into the backseat, clutching mine. Ten minutes later, we were in the home we had bought especially for this occasion, just one month earlier.

I had barely slept since Henry's birth. I was up all night feeding him, holding him, and obsessively watching for any signs that he was turning blue. That first week, we spent a lot of time in waiting rooms and hospitals as we visited our growing list of doctors: Henry's pediatrician, his cardiologist, a geneticist. Each day, we learned a little more about his condition and fell a lot more in love with him. During one visit, Dr. Kenneth Rosenbaum, the head of genetics at Children's National Medical Center, explained to us that multiple birth defects—like Henry's relatively low birth weight, extra thumb, and heart defect—are often linked to a broader syndrome. Much to our relief, he quickly eliminated many horrifying possibilities. The only test result we were awaiting was for something so rare Dr. Rosenbaum didn't even bother to tell us its name.

The name, it turns out, is Fanconi anemia.

"*F*anconi anemia."

"I'm sorry?" I heard Allen say into the phone two weeks later. We were lying in bed together late on a Friday afternoon in early November, catching a quick respite between feedings, diaper changes, laundry, and doctors' appointments. Henry was peacefully sleeping in the bassinet next to our bed. "Can you please repeat that?"

I didn't know this at the time, having never heard of Fanconi anemia before, but those two little words were about to wipe out all the dreams I'd ever held for my family in a matter of seconds. Later, when I thought about that moment, it's not the hearing of the words that I remember as much as the moment right before it. The moment when it was only his thumb and heart. Those problems, I'd learn, were easy to fix. Like many new moms, I had a stack of books on my night table that promised to help me navigate my way through parenthood, but none of them prepared me for Fanconi anemia.

Henry's Favorite Things

- Jack
  - Blowing bubbles
    - Driving Papa Sy's Farmall tractor
  - Yoda, especially in the final scene of
    Star Wars Episode II: Attack of the Clones
- Pony rides
  - Squidward's comment to SpongeBob: "Could
    you keep it down? I'm trying to be boring."
- Root-beer-flavored anesthesia

3

The Wonder Years

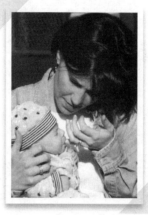

Henry tries to swallow me whole

*G*rowing up outside of Washington, DC, the mantra in my home was "There's always room for one more." Our house was a meeting place where neighborhood kids, family, and friends of all ages gathered for food, fun, and conversation. Our pantry was stocked with cookie-making ingredients, and our garage with balls, skis, bikes, stilts, and other suburban accoutrements. Our days were filled with public school, visits to parks and museums, and hikes on the C & O Canal. Our nights initially featured Red Rover and Kick the Can and, eventually, late-night excursions to the Tastee Diner in Bethesda, Maryland, in my 1947 Willy's Jeep or my friends' Duster or Pinto. The rules in my family were simple: Be honest, treat others the way you wanted to be treated, give back to the community, work hard, be prepared, and enjoy. When, from time to time, things didn't go our way and Abby, Andrew, or I would exclaim, "It's not fair," my dad, Sy Strongin, a labor arbitrator by trade, would answer, "Life's not fair." I listened, but the truth is, I didn't believe him.

I'm not sure whether it was out of fear of being average or just my nature, but as far back as I can remember, I had always hovered around the extremes, at least for a suburban good girl. I would run ten miles in a stretch and then eat a pound of M&M's. One summer I won honor camper and after another, I was asked not to return to sleep-away camp due to a series of episodes involving capsized boats and bras up the flagpole. I was captain of the Bethesda–Chevy Chase High School field hockey team and on the homecoming court. I held the esteemed position of being one of two women to participate in the University of Michigan's first-ever Nude Mile in 1986 but took comfort in the predictability of living an adult life that mirrored the one I had as a child: a life based around family, trust, and love.

For Allen and me, it wasn't love at first sight. The first time we met, Allen Goldberg and I were each out on a date with someone else. But by the end of the night as we drove out of the Tower Records parking lot in downtown Washington, listening to the words of U2's *Rattle and Hum* as loud as Allen's VW Golf stereo would allow, a friendship was born.

It was 1988. Allen was twenty-six, Jewish, good-looking in an unintentional way, smart, employed, and fun. He was tall, redheaded, and had a pair of dimples I could sink my fingers into. Having grown up in the Washington area and never straying too far from home, Allen knew all its secrets, like the intimate and romantic wine cellar at the now-closed Dolce Finale in Woodley Park that sat about four people, and Joe's Record Paradise in Rockville, which stocked bootlegged albums and featured little-known local artists. Allen loved music, and his record collection rivaled mine.

He's never been a paint-the-face kind of fan, but like many Washingtonians, Allen rooted for the Redskins. For him, fall and winter Sundays were game-focused, and the general mood was determined by wins or losses. He threw parties that strained the square footage of his Northwest DC apartment, as well as his neighbors' nerves. Allen's ability to enjoy everything was contagious. Even McDonald's recognized this, featuring him in a national advertising campaign in which he exclaimed, "Excellent!" in response to a question about what he'd say if they told him their burgers were only seventy-nine cents. "Excellent" was what Allen would say about most things, and that made him the kind of guy I wanted to be around.

At the time, Allen worked at a DC-based national trade association, and I was a communications consultant. Allen hired me to plan a tribute dinner for his mentor and retiring boss, George W. Koch, CEO of the Grocery Manufacturers of America, whose daughter was afflicted with colitis. The event was a fund-raiser for what is now the Crohn's and Colitis Foundation of America. I'm still not sure if Allen hired me based on my credentials, my girl-next-door appeal, or some combination of the two, but the event was a tremendous personal and professional success for us. It also set the standard for what would become a lifetime partnership built on loyalty, the importance of family, good deeds, and good parties.

There was something comfortable and familiar about Allen. Maybe it was the fact that we grew up five miles from each other in the Chevy Chase and Potomac, Maryland, suburbs of Washington. We were both children of professionals and grandchildren of immigrants, coming of age insulated by the suburbs. We were reluctant dog walkers; got shuttled to and fro in station wagons; camped in West Virginia; and spent summers at the Delaware shore. Growing up, we were both extremely fortunate to have dodged the trend and trauma of parental divorce, the worries of financial instability, and the horror of significant health problems.

I was twenty-three, and Allen was my best friend. For four years, we shared beach-house rentals; went to rock concerts at the Bayou, Grog and Tankard, Wolf Trap, and other venues; took road trips to New York City and New Orleans; danced to reggae at Kilimanjaro in Washington, rock and funk at the Bottle & Cork in Dewey Beach, Delaware, and zydeco at the New Orleans Jazz Fest. We dated other people, but every six months or so, Allen would point out the obvious: We were made for each other. But I couldn't see why we would let romance ruin what we had.

One morning in February 1992, I woke up with a start and realized that Allen was right. I called him and asked him on a date that transformed us from friends into everything he's since become to me. He was as good a boyfriend as he was a friend. He listened to what I had to say. He paid attention to my interests. He took care of me while respecting and admiring my independence. He made me feel special.

Four years after we met, I beat Allen at Battleship. It was pouring and cold, and we were at my parents' house on the Chesapeake Bay outside Annapolis, Maryland. I played the trick where you cluster the ships and make it nearly impossible for your opponent to figure out where one ship ends and the other begins. Allen protested that after Pearl Harbor no one does that in real life, but I did. After the game, Allen suggested we walk down to the water. Despite my insistence that warm soup and a hot fire held greater appeal, I agreed.

We went for a walk and came home engaged.

· · ·

As I was preparing to get married in the spring of 1993, my friends were busy preparing a proper bachelorette party for me. In high school, my friends Erica Antonelli, Laura Subrin, and Becca Knox and I had started our own little clique, which we called BOA (Bitches of America). We had business cards printed and thought it was all very cool. Of course, "cool" for us meant that we were good students who engaged in innocent fun, like streaking naked along the Beltway on the afternoon of our SATs. For our sixteenth birthdays, we had sweatshirts made up: black ones with BOA printed in white capital letters on the front. We'd wear them to meet up with our boyfriends at the all-night Tastee Diner. We had a blast.

After college, most of us returned to Washington. Erica, Becca, and I—as well as other women we'd met in college and through friends—began to meet once a month for dinner at the Pines of Rome restaurant in downtown Bethesda, not far from where our teenage antics had occurred, and where one of us had had her sweet-sixteen party. It was a classic Italian place with red-and-white tablecloths and candles stuck in large wine bottles on the tables. We'd drink house red out of small juice glasses and begin every meal with a large white pizza for the table. We called ourselves the Ladies of the Pines.

It was here that my friends met to organize my bachelorette party, and a few weeks before my wedding day, the Ladies of the Pines arrived at my parents' house to pick me up. On the hood of the minivan they rented was a huge banner: DESTINATION ANYWHERE. We blasted Bruce Springsteen, Elvis Costello, Billy Bragg, and U2 and drove to Atlantic City, where we spent most of the night laughing, reminiscing, and dancing in our hotel room.

On May 15, 1993, I married my best friend. It was a perfect day, unseasonably warm and sunny at Washington Harbour on the

Potomac River. When we broke the ceremonial glass and kissed as husband and wife, the 230 guests, as well as the hundreds of other diners and boaters, all cheered.

We never talked about whether we would have kids, because it was a given that we would. The only question was when. Like many Ashkenazi Jews, we underwent genetic testing to determine whether we were carriers of Tay Sachs, a fatal genetic disease in the Jewish population, and the only one for which testing was available at the time. We both tested negative. Since neither of us had any history of genetic disease in our families, we were unconcerned about passing along anything deadly to our children. We just wondered if they would be redheads with green eyes, and tall and thin like Allen; or brown-haired with brown eyes, and short and olive-skinned like me. We were pretty clear on one fact: They'd probably be good dancers.

"I'm sorry, can you spell it?" Allen was now saying as I lay beside him, reading the notes he was jotting on a scrap of paper. *Fanconi anemia. Rare. Fatal? Henry.*

The first things I learned about Fanconi anemia were that it causes a bunch of birth defects and it has the impossible-to-accept label "fatal." Over time, I came to know the truth about Fanconi anemia. It's shit and piss and blood and agonizing pain. It's twenty-one or twenty-four medications a day, anesthesia, surgery, infection, malnutrition. It's hoping your child will be lucky enough to make it to the first day of kindergarten. It's interminable days and sleepless nights without a break; fear; loneliness; desperation. It's the possibility of death, each day. It's longing for an escape, and the awful, horrible realization that the only escape is death. It's knowing that death would be far, far worse. It's thoughts of throwing dirt on your boy's coffin. It's not knowing how you are going to live without him. It's having to live without him.

I'm glad I didn't know all that at the time. It was way too much for a new mom to comprehend.

. . .

Allen hung up the phone, and I leaned over and scooped Henry out of the bassinet and into my arms. There are three bedrooms upstairs in our rowhouse, and Henry's room was in the back. It had a wall of windows that filled the room with sunlight. Everything was a pretty, comforting blue: his crib and dresser, and the walls, to which we had affixed a sweet wallpaper border of a beach scene. For the first few weeks after his birth, though, he slept near us. I held Henry tight to my chest to shield him from those menacing words that threatened to steal our happiness. Allen, meanwhile, went to the computer and typed the foreign name into an Internet search engine.

Named for the Swiss physician who first identified it in 1927, Fanconi anemia (FA) is an inherited anemia, passed along from parents to their children. It is a recessive disorder, meaning that both parents have to carry and then pass along a defect, or mutation, in the same FA gene in order to have a child afflicted with FA. In other words, Allen and I had unknowingly given this disease to Henry at the same time we had given him brown hair, brown eyes, and the absolute cutest dimples I had ever seen. Researchers estimate that one out of every three hundred people is an FA carrier; but among Ashkenazi Jews like Allen and me, the carrier frequency is approximately one out of every ninety. By the year Henry was born, approximately one thousand people had been diagnosed with FA worldwide, and Allen and I didn't know a single one of them.

Some of the websites we visited used the word "fatal" to describe FA. Others used "often fatal," and some even "usually fatal." I would have given everything I had for a "rarely fatal" or "seldom fatal." But no matter how hard or how often we searched, those words never appeared.

The first few weeks at home, I tried to figure out how to breast-feed and change Henry's diaper, and get his little arms into his undershirt, while recovering from my C-section. I struggled to absorb all of the news we were being forced to understand. He might turn blue any moment. He would definitely need open-heart surgery in the next few months.

He could die before kindergarten?

My mom called a friend and got the name of a pediatric hematologist, whom Allen and I called that very night. In addition to giving us the names of experts, the hematologist planted a critical seed of hope. Although Fanconi anemia was still considered a fatal genetic disease, she explained that the dismal death rates reported were out-of-date, as science was advancing and with it, the chance that Henry could survive.

The day after Henry was diagnosed with FA, we visited Dr. Rosenbaum at Children's National Medical Center, who opened his office on the weekend to explain everything he knew about FA and to give us the names and phone numbers of the very best specialists. He also gave us a quick genetics course, explaining that Allen and I were each carriers because at least one of each of our parents was a carrier and had passed it along to us at birth. Through blood tests we soon learned that in our case, each of our mothers was a carrier. Being a carrier isn't a concern as long as your spouse isn't a carrier. Since neither my father nor Allen's was a carrier, our parents would never have a child with Fanconi anemia. However, when one carrier (Allen) marries another (me), with each pregnancy, we had a 25 percent chance of having a baby with the disease; a 25 percent chance of having a baby who is healthy and not a carrier; and a 50 percent chance that the baby would be healthy, but a carrier like us. In other words, Allen and I were unknowingly playing Russian roulette with our children's lives.

There are at least thirteen FA genes or complementation groups. FA-A, FA-C (Henry's type), and FA-G account for nearly 85 percent of all cases. The disease occurs equally in males and females, and is found in all ethnic groups, although the percentage of Jews who have FA is higher than the percentage of Jews in the general population, making it a disproportionately Jewish disease. The median age for the onset of bone-marrow failure is seven, and the average life expectancy is twenty-two years, but the actual life span of any one individual can be quite different from the average. Kids like Henry with FA-C tend to have the most severe birth defects and earlier onset of bone-marrow failure. They also have the poorest bone-marrow-transplant survival rates—or the highest death rate—following a transplant.

Henry's geneticist first suspected FA because of Henry's relatively low birth weight, extra thumb, and heart defect, which were not a coincidence. However, we learned that doctors usually fail to diagnose FA at birth, since few of them have experience with the disease, and also because there are a multitude of possible birth defects, it presents differently in different kids. Even identical twins born with FA can have differing birth defects. Some babies are missing thumbs or kidneys, have malformed digestive tracts, or have hearing loss. Some have no birth defects at all. The majority of children are diagnosed only after a series of infections or nosebleeds lead to a blood test that reveals aplastic anemia or bone-marrow failure.

Aplastic anemia, a condition in which the bone marrow does not produce enough red cells, white cells, or platelets, almost always develops in children with FA. It compromises the body's ability to fight infection, causes spontaneous bleeding and exhaustion, and ultimately leads to death. The most successful treatment for aplastic anemia is a hematopoietic stem-cell transplant with blood stem cells derived from the bone marrow—commonly referred to as a bone-marrow transplant.

Although successful stem-cell transplants can cure aplastic anemia, Fanconi patients also have a much higher risk of other cancers—such as acute myeloid leukemia, squamous cell carcinoma of the head and neck, and cervical and liver cancer—than the general population. So patients who are lucky enough to survive a stem-cell transplant, while unlikely to develop leukemia, are likely to face a subsequent diagnosis of one cancer or another, and must endure the medical challenges again and again.

Among the doctor's referrals was an organization, the Fanconi Anemia Research Fund (FARF), founded by Lynn and Dave Frohnmayer—parents of five children, three of whom were born with FA—who had since devoted their lives to raising money and funding research. FARF also provides much-needed information and support to families who, like ours, unwittingly joined a club of which no one would choose to be a member. From our first conversation, Lynn and Dave provided us with comfort that we were not alone in our fight to save Henry. They also gave us an abundance of information about Fanconi anemia, and their friendship.

When we got the news about FA in early November 1995, my sister, Abby, had a one-week-old daughter, Rachel, and an eighteen-month-old son, Michael; my brother, Andrew, and his wife were expecting their first baby in five months; and Allen's sister, Jennifer, had a one-year-old, Hannah. No one knew who was and wasn't a carrier or who might already or soon have a child with a deadly disease. They visited geneticists and hugged their kids a little tighter as they anxiously awaited the test results. In every case, our family members were eventually told that they were lucky enough to have genes that did not foretell the premature death of their children.

Allen and I spent the first few months of Henry's life shopping for diapers, onesies, a breast pump, hematologists, cardiologists, and pediatric surgeons. We interviewed doctors in Washington; New York City; Hackensack, New Jersey; and Boston. We settled on a cardiologist in Washington, a hematologist in Hackensack, a cardiac surgeon and a hand surgeon in Boston, and a Medela Pump In Style breast pump.

Henry, meanwhile, spent the first few weeks and months of his life doing the things that babies do. He learned to turn his head from side to side, roll over from his tummy to his back, play with his fingers and toes, and smile. He smiled when he heard my voice. He smiled when Allen or I held him. He smiled when we listened to good music. I was the first of the Ladies of the Pines to have a child, and Erica, Becca, and my neighbor Debbie Blum—also a member and a pregnant one at that—adored Henry. They stopped by all the time. Erica was playing with him one day in our family room, making faces and singing to him. Staring down at him, she exclaimed adoringly, "Laurie, this kid's smile is too big for his face!"

Abby, Rachel, Henry, and I spent a lot of time together those first few months. I'd strap Henry in the BabyBjörn and walk over to Abby's house, about a mile away, and we would head to Georgetown for coffee or lunch. Henry was happy, easy, and incredibly adorable. And most important, his defective heart did what it needed to do and he never turned blue, defying the predicted path and reassuring me that I could trust Allen's optimism.

And proving to us that Henry was extraordinary.

Henry's Favorite Things

- Batman
  - Cal Ripken
    - Collecting baseball cards
  - Traversing the monkey bars
- Going to Spring Training
  - Flushing saline through his own IV lines
- Chocolate-chip pancakes

4

MAKING CHOICES

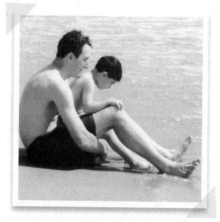

Allen and Henry ponder the surf in Bethany
Beach, Delaware

ong before the words "Fanconi anemia" entered my lexis, I
had dreamed of having three kids, and always pictured myself surrounded by boys. My mother, Pat Strongin, is a great mom and a
great role model. She is young at heart, active, and full of life; growing up, she took us kids biking, camping, swimming, and horseback
riding. With her boundless energy and joy, her popularity extended
well beyond the family to include all my friends who spent countless

hours hanging out in our childhood home. Even Allen later admitted that after meeting my mom, he decided to marry me. He saw signs of me in her and found her to be "really cool . . . for a mom." My dad, meanwhile, has always been the Godfather of our family. He smokes cigars, likes a good glass of scotch, reads voraciously, thinks about things, and doles out instructions and wisdom. He is one of the most adventurous men I know. I had always imagined that I'd be the same type of parent to my kids that they had been to Abby, Andrew, and me: fun, love-filled, supportive, and completely comfortable with mayhem. I imagined a house, yard, and garage filled with sports equipment; a kitchen with plentiful snacks and family dinners; a playroom with games, drums, guitars, and a pinball machine; vacations at the beach; and baseball games on the weekends. Loud, crazy, spontaneous fun.

Allen and I wanted to have several children, but Fanconi anemia made family planning about a whole lot more than love and sex. All of a sudden, it was a complex puzzle of genes, statistical probability, prenatal testing, and life-or-death decisions. It wasn't just about creating life but about avoiding certain death. The very best prenatal care might be a good weapon against some diseases, like spina bifida, but it is useless against Fanconi anemia. Because Allen and I are both FA carriers, there was an uncomfortably high chance that we could have another baby with the disease. Although there was a 75 percent chance that our next baby would be healthy, our life experience taught us that statistics are predictions, not promises. After all, the chance of our having a baby with FA was 1 in 30,000. Once you hit a number like that, you stop taking comfort in the remoteness of a chance that something bad could happen.

Through conversations with FARF leadership and our growing list of doctors, as well as our own research, Allen and I understood that Henry would need open-heart surgery at around six months of age and a bone-marrow transplant probably by the time he turned five. Though I was scared to death at the prospect of open-heart surgery, I understood that the bone-marrow transplant was the real challenge. Our best hope—if not our only one—that Henry would survive a transplant was if we could find a perfectly matched stem-cell donor. The only perfectly matched donors are siblings.

At this time, in 1995, bone-marrow transplants from perfectly matched sibling donors had reported success rates of 85 percent. This meant that if we had another baby who did not inherit Fanconi anemia and whose bone marrow was compatible with Henry's, then Henry would probably survive. When the baby was born, doctors could collect its umbilical-cord blood through a painless and harmless procedure, transplant it to Henry, and silence the most lethal threat to his life.

In contrast, the success rate for a bone-marrow transplant from an unrelated donor—someone other than a sibling—was around 18 percent, meaning that without a sibling donor, Henry would probably die. At the time, no one with his type of FA had ever survived a transplant without a perfectly matched sibling donor.

What this meant for us, in the simplest terms, was that Henry's life depended on our having another baby with two critical characteristics: the baby had to be Fanconi anemia–free, and needed to be a human leukocyte antigen (HLA) match to Henry. HLA, also known as histocompatibility antigens, are genes that recognize whether a cell is foreign to the body. Any cell possessing an individual's HLA type is recognized as belonging to that person, whereas a cell with a different HLA type is identified as an invader. Like all invaders, these cells are unwelcome, and the resulting internal battle can cause mild to great bodily harm and even death.

HLA type is used to determine the compatibility of bone marrow, kidney, liver, pancreas, and heart for transplantation from one person to another. Compatibility between organ donor and recipient is judged by the number of HLA antigens found in the donor that are shared by the recipient. In 1995, bone-marrow-transplant compatibility was determined by six HLA antigens, including two each of HLA-A, HLA-B, and HLA-DR. Everyone acquires one set of three from each parent. Today, the testing is more sophisticated and the best donor would share eight antigens, which include HLA-C. The very best organ donor for Henry would be someone with the *exact* same HLA antigens. HLA type is inherited, and that is why siblings have the greatest likelihood of being perfectly matched at the HLA antigens and why they are therefore the ideal donors.

Nothing was guaranteed. Because, like Fanconi anemia, HLA type is genetic, the chance of another baby being a perfect HLA match to Henry was just 25 percent. But Fanconi anemia further diminished those odds. If the sibling also had FA, he or she would not only be disqualified as a stem-cell donor but would also suffer from the disease, would probably experience significant birth defects, and eventually need a transplant from a healthy sibling. The probability that we would have a healthy baby who would also be an HLA match to Henry—the ideal-case scenario—was merely 18.75 percent, or one-quarter of the 75 percent chance that the baby would be healthy.

In other words, it was a long shot.

Allen and I talked a lot about having another child, weighing all of our options. The only absolute guarantee that our future children wouldn't have FA was if we adopted or did artificial insemination, using a donated sperm or donated eggs. Or, of course, we could decide to stop having children altogether. At the time, our inherent optimism combined with our determination not to let Fanconi anemia dictate every move, and our deep desire for more children, blinded us to those alternatives.

I thought a lot about my ability to provide not just a life for a new baby, but a good life, even in the worst of circumstances. We knew it was a serious decision to have another child who was certain to experience extreme hardship and the potential loss of a sibling. I talked with Allen, perhaps more than he would have liked, about all the fears and uncertainties I felt.

"What are we doing? Are we being irresponsible, risking having another child with FA?" I asked him over dinner at Lebanese Taverna, our date-night destination; and again, a few days later, as we drove home from a visit to New York, where we had been shopping for doctors. "I know I want to have more kids, but our life is going to be so hard and I'm scared to bring another child into it. It's not like this baby is asking to be born," I said. "We're going to bring him or her into a family filled with lots of love, to be sure, but also the guarantee of so much hardship with Henry's illness. I just don't know if that is the right thing to do."

Allen listened, but he didn't share my concerns.

"Laurie, you don't have to take all that on right now. Henry is going to be fine. And our next baby is going to be healthy. And lucky. You know how much we love Henry? That's how much we're going to love the next one, too," he responded.

In the end, I felt strongly that choosing to have another child meant that Allen and I were committing to surviving, even if Henry didn't, and it wasn't long before we arrived at our decision: We were going to have another child. Although we hoped our second child would be an HLA match to Henry, our main concern was that he or she would be healthy.

A few days later, during a walk through the neighborhood with Henry, I confided in my mom. "Allen and I talked about it. We're going to have another baby after Henry's heart surgery is over. I really want to have more kids," I explained. "I don't want to let Fanconi take that away from me too."

"Laurie, I'm so happy to hear that," my mom said. "I *want* you to have more kids. You should. You were meant to be a mother. You're a great mother. And any child of yours is one lucky kid."

"But I'm scared," I confessed. "I don't know what I'll do if that child has Fanconi, if I could live through that again. Knowing what's ahead of us, and what Henry faces . . . it's so hard."

My mom stopped walking and took my hand in hers. "Laurie, you will do whatever you have to do. When you were just a year and a half old, Grandma said to me, 'That one has something special,' and you do."

Before I got pregnant again, I needed to survive Henry's open-heart surgery. Actually, I needed Henry to survive Henry's open-heart surgery. I knew that I wouldn't be able to sleep or eat while I sat in a waiting room worrying about whether Henry would make it through his time on a heart-lung machine and the recovery from his surgery. If I did get pregnant right away, I wanted to make sure our new baby was developing in the healthiest prenatal environment possible. Also, I knew I couldn't simultaneously handle the trauma of Henry's heart surgery while waiting for, and processing, prenatal test results that would tell us if our second child also had Fanconi anemia, which could be determined at the end of the first trimester.

Henry's open-heart surgery was scheduled for April 2, 1996, with Dr. Richard Jonas at Boston Children's Hospital. The days leading up to the trip, I packed Henry's stuff, asked our neighbors Rich and Jill Lane to pick up our mail and keep an eye on the house, called Erica and Becca to tell them I'd miss that month's Ladies of the Pines meeting, and desperately hoped for the best. A few days after we arrived, my parents, Allen's parents, and Abby joined us in Boston, where we had been meeting with doctors and preparing for the surgery. We had been told that we wouldn't be allowed to spend the night at the hospital, so we checked into the Best Western Hotel immediately adjacent to it. The day before Henry's surgery, I took the advice of another mother, a friend's cousin whose son had endured the same procedure at the same hospital. She had encouraged us to visit the pediatric cardiac intensive care prior to his surgery, thinking that we needed to know what, exactly, we were in for.

Walking in there for the first time was as scary as hell. There were no private rooms, just curtains separating kids—about ten of them—all in perilous situations and fighting for their lives. The nursing station was central so that the staff could be at a child's bedside in a moment. Dazed, weary parents talked in hushed tones, and the kids were in drug-induced comas, resting while their hearts healed. It was an eerie quiet, interrupted only by the frightening, panicked clamor of pumps, machines, alarms.

On the morning of his surgery, we brought Henry to the hospital before the sun rose and sat with him until the anesthesiologists approached. They tickled him. They smiled at him. And then before we knew it, they were gone. With Henry.

We sat in the waiting room, waiting. Surrounded by untouched food, unopened magazines and books, our parents and my sister, we just sat. There was nothing to talk about other than the obvious, and we saw no point talking about that. So we sat in silence, and we waited.

With each major step, a nurse came to inform us of Henry's progress. He's under anesthesia. He's on oxygen. I was so scared, I honestly didn't know if I would get through it. When the nurse came to tell us he was on the heart-lung machine, all I heard was: *His heart isn't beating. Their hands are in there. They're touching his heart.* But then she returned, a few hours after it had begun, to tell us that he was off the heart-lung machine; that his heart was working again. He was being brought to the recovery room. *He is alive!* I don't know if those words actually passed my lips, but the way I remember it, I yelled it more loudly and joyfully than anything I had ever shouted before.

Even if I had spent months in that pediatric intensive care unit trying to get comfortable with the images and the reality of what Henry would have to endure, nothing would have prepared me for what I saw when Henry first came out of surgery. It was terrifying. His whole body was swollen and his skin looked like it was made of plastic. White surgical tape held his oxygen mask in place. Dozens of tubes ran into and out of his body. The bandages covering his chest were soaked in blood. It was, as of that day, the most horrifying image I'd ever seen.

I leaned over his tiny body. "Please get through this," I whispered to him. "I know it's only been five months, but I can't remember my life before you."

Henry spent the next few days in his hospital bed, between two curtains that we could close for some privacy. He wore nothing but a diaper and lay completely motionless in a drug-induced paralysis. We could not hold him or hug him. We could merely stand there and stare and hope he'd wake up. There were lots of monitors beeping and flashing, recording his oxygen level and heart rate and blood gasses and, I imagine, other stuff. I studied the numbers, the charts, and the levels, trying to understand what they meant, what they could tell me. Hoping, desperately, that he was improving.

On the second morning, Allen and I arrived at the ICU and saw that the incubator next to Henry's was empty. I asked the nurse on duty what had happened to the newborn baby who was there the night before. It was a stupid question, perhaps, or at least an obvious one. The bed was stripped of its sheets, the medical equipment shut off. The nurse told us the boy's name: Henry. I felt a sharp pang of sadness for the tiny boy's parents, for his unlived life.

Over the next few days, my breasts ached from the desire to feed our Henry, but my milk had dried up because I was unwilling to leave his bedside to pump milk that he was too weak to drink and that would just be thrown away. For the time being, his nutrition was delivered through one of the many tubes pumping fluids into and out of his tiny body. Were it not for the machines that indicated to the contrary, I would have thought he was dead.

We stayed as long as we could each day, until the nurses told us to leave. They'd gently shoo us out the door, and we'd stumble next door to the hotel, lay down on top of the scratchy, polyester comforter, clutching the pager they'd given us in case something went wrong.

But nothing went wrong. In fact, everything went right. Ten days later, Henry was well enough to go home. Dr. Jonas informed us that the surgery had gone perfectly. Henry was not in pain, and the fear that he could turn blue was erased from our lives. Walking back into our home, with our heart-healthy son wrapped in the blanket my mom had knitted and presented to me at a baby shower that seemed like a lifetime ago, was definitely one of the best days I'd had in what felt like a very, very long time.

The fact that Dr. Hougen had been right about the 99 percent success rate associated with Henry's surgery greatly boosted our confidence in the team of doctors we had begun to assemble to treat his FA. It also made me feel more comfortable about the idea of returning to work. Four months before Henry was born, I had earned my master's of social work (MSW) at Catholic University of America, giving a graduation speech to my fellow students about the critical need and our obligation to help repair the world we'd inherited. Afterward, I accepted a job at a national nonprofit housing organization, Neighborhood Reinvestment Corporation, to focus my attention on increasing the availability of affordable housing. That they hired me while I was clearly pregnant was predictive of the way they treated me when I became the mother of a beautiful, very ill, little boy.

After my maternity leave ended, we entrusted six-month-old Henry to the care of Allen's parents, Phyllis and Ted, affectionately known as Grandma and Pop Pop Teddy, and I returned to work several days a week. I had mixed feelings about this. Henry was totally healthy by then. Other than monthly tests to check his complete blood counts (CBCs), which evaluated his overall health and attempted to detect a wide range of disorders, including anemia, infection, and leukemia; and a semiannual bone-marrow aspiration and biopsy to check on the progress of his disease, he was a normal, spunky kid. But I still found it hard to leave him each morning. Every day on our way to work, I'd remind Allen not to let me quit my job. I knew I just needed time to get used to being back at work. I always told myself that 99 percent of women in the world had to work to earn money (a statistic I'm quite sure I made up), and so I too would work, and not feel sorry for myself. Plus, I honestly loved my job, my work, and my colleagues. They were among the most supportive, terrific group of people I knew, and I also felt strongly about the work my organization did to help house low- and moderate-income families.

Henry, as mellow as he was, probably had much less conflicted feelings than I about the matter. He adored Grandma and Pop Pop Teddy, who would make the twenty-minute drive to our house every morning. Ted would go to work while Phyllis spent the day with Henry. She had been recently diagnosed with malignant melanoma and felt a special bond to her grandson, whose constant smile threatened to make her forget her own plight. She loved to read to him, *Babar* especially, and afterward, the two of them would gather on the couch to watch *Wallace & Gromit* cartoons.

When we returned home at the end of the day, before Allen or I could even take our coats off, Phyllis would convey, in painstaking detail, all of Henry's extraordinary accomplishments over the last eight hours. One evening, as I listened to her recall stories of their trip to the park, and the people's hearts he had won over, I looked over and noticed that he happened to be wearing yet another new, hand-knit sweater with little woolly sheep that she had just made for him. We were incredibly lucky to have such a wonderful mother nearby who would volunteer to babysit our son and relish every moment of it.

In May 1996, not long after Henry turned six months old, we found out that I was pregnant. Like any couple trying to become pregnant, we were euphoric. But fear and uncertainty quickly crept in. Instead of calling our parents to share the good news, our first phone calls were to our doctors.

A few hours after learning that I was pregnant, I was sitting in the dining room when the phone rang. It was Dr. Arleen Auerbach, a preeminent Fanconi researcher. Everyone with a child diagnosed with FA knows to call Dr. Auerbach first. Toiling behind the beautiful gates of Rockefeller University's ivy-drenched castle on New York City's Upper East Side, Dr. Auerbach, who manages the International Fanconi Anemia Registry, knows nearly all one thousand FA patients and their families. When Dr. Rosenbaum saw Henry's extra thumb at birth, a defect occasionally associated with Fanconi anemia, he sent a blood sample to Dr. Auerbach, and it was she who had diagnosed Henry with the disease.

We spoke for a long time, and when I finally hung up the phone with her, I felt stunned. And elated.

"Allen!" I yelled to my husband, who was upstairs. "Can you come down here? Like right now!"

A few minutes later, he walked into the sun-filled dining room, where I sat, still in my pajamas, the phone in my hands.

"What's wrong?" he said. "You all right?" He sat down across from me.

"Listen," I said, trying to compose myself. "What would you say if I told you that we could get pregnant and know that our baby was going to be healthy?"

"Well, isn't it a little late for that?" asked Allen.

"Seriously, just tell me. What would you say?"

"I'd say sign us up," he said, confirming the obvious.

"What if we could also know that the baby was a bone-marrow match for Henry?" I added.

"I'd say we'd found the golden ticket," he replied.

"Well, I think we just did. It's called PGD."

As Dr. Auerbach had explained to me, PGD, or preimplantation genetic diagnosis, was a cutting-edge, newly available process that could allow us to know at the moment of pregnancy that our next baby was both healthy and HLA-matched to Henry. Dr. Mark Hughes, the chief of the Section on Reproductive and Prenatal Genetics in the Diagnostic Development Branch of the National Center for Human Genome Research at the National Institutes of Health; professor of medicine, pediatrics, and OB/GYN at Georgetown University Medical Center; and a pioneer in the field of reproductive genetics, specifically in single-cell genetic analysis, had figured out a way to combine in vitro fertilization with genetic testing conducted prior to embryo transfer. PGD would enable us to identify and implant an artificially conceived embryo that was not only healthy, but who could also be Henry's savior. By collecting this healthy baby's umbilical cord blood at birth and transplanting the stem cells to Henry, our baby could cure Henry's blood disease.

"Preimplantation genetic diagnosis." Three words that, strung together, are easily passed over like so many medical terms that can be mistaken for a foreign language. Individually the words are powerful. "Preimplantation." Before implantation. Before becoming my baby. Insurance against ever having to consider abortion. "Genetic." Inherited. In this case, a disease best expelled from our gene pool.

"Diagnosis." Certainty. A guarantee that Fanconi anemia could never again threaten to destroy one of my babies. Together these words formed a profound source of hope and dominated our life. And the shorthand, PGD, became part of our family vocabulary.

Dr. Hughes had used PGD in the past to screen embryos for fatal childhood diseases like sickle cell anemia and cystic fibrosis, enabling parents to know at the outset that their babies would not be born with a disease. But neither he—nor anyone else in the world—had ever used PGD to find a perfect HLA match, from whom umbilical cord stem cells could be harvested and thus save a sibling.

"In other words, we'd be the first?" Allen asked me.

"Apparently so."

"Wait. Let me get this straight. We'd be the *first, ever, anywhere*?"

Preimplantation genetic diagnosis involves the biopsy of one or two cells from an eight-cell embryo, typically on the third day following egg retrieval, as part of an in vitro fertilization cycle. The biopsy is performed in a laboratory by making an opening in the outer "shell" of the embryo with a micropipette. One or two cells are extracted through this opening in an extremely delicate procedure. Once the embryo has been biopsied, it takes about forty-eight hours for the genetic testing to be completed before the embryo, which remains in a lab and continues to develop to the blastocyst stage, must be transferred to the woman's uterus to be able to produce a viable pregnancy.

The extracted cell(s) are analyzed to determine the genetic composition of the embryo. These tests can determine the presence of Down's syndrome or trisomy 21, among other chromosomal abnormalities. Testing can also be done for couples known to carry diseases caused by a single gene abnormality, such as FA. To determine whether an embryo has FA, a technique known as a polymerase chain reaction (PCR) is used to replicate the targeted gene. These copies are examined for evidence of a particular DNA sequence that reveals the presence or absence of FA. The results of preimplantation genetic diagnosis are used to inform the selection of embryos for transfer to a woman's uterus, enabling her to begin her pregnancy with the knowledge that her baby will not possess the life-threatening childhood disease.

It has been more than a decade since physicians like Dr. Hughes have used PGD for disease prevention. Today, approximately one thousand babies have been born using this technique. But in 1996, when we began talking with Drs. Auerbach and Hughes, PGD had never been used to test for HLA type or any other trait that was not a matter of survival to the embryo being tested.

Dr. Hughes had agreed to offer PGD with HLA typing to FA families who met several very specific criteria. First of all, the mother had to be under thirty-five years old; at the time I was thirty-one. Younger mothers typically produce more eggs in the process of in vitro fertilization and therefore have a greater likelihood of success. They also have a lower risk of producing eggs with abnormal chromosomes. In addition, Dr. Hughes would work only with families who had already expressed an interest in having additional children, meaning that the baby born through this technology would be wanted, independent of its ability to save its sibling's life. My current pregnancy was proof that we were determined to continue to grow our family, despite Fanconi anemia. Last, the family had to have the FA-C, IVS4 Fanconi mutation, because it was the only type of FA for which the gene had been discovered, and therefore was the only type of FA that could be diagnosed through PGD.

Allen, Henry, and I were one of only two families who met the criteria.

If we pursued PGD, Allen and I would be entering completely uncharted territory. As the first people in the world to use this technology for this purpose, there was no precedent, no books or articles to read, and no support groups. There were no established ethical guidelines or government or industry regulation of PGD. There would be no guarantees except that the unknown held possibilities that otherwise eluded us. Henry's open-heart surgery was behind us, but a bone-marrow transplant with a dismal survival rate awaited. I was in my first trimester of pregnancy, with eight weeks to go before a prenatal test could tell us whether the child I was carrying had FA. PGD was our lifeline out of this horror.

We would wait for the results of prenatal testing that would determine whether the baby I was carrying was healthy. If so, regardless of HLA type, we would continue the pregnancy. As first-time parents of a baby newly recovered from open-heart surgery with inconceivable hardship on the horizon, we didn't have the luxury of time, energy, or imagination to figure out what we would do if our second baby was struck with FA. But we were grateful to know that we had choices.

Allen and I carefully considered the ethical implications of PGD. We had so many things to consider and so little information. We were determined to protect and advocate for Henry, and for our future children, while also honoring our values and those of the broader community in which we lived.

For more than half a century, prenatal diagnosis through procedures like amniocentesis and chorionic villus sampling has enabled couples to screen their fetuses for genetic disorders. Since that time, couples like us have faced the difficult dilemma as to whether to proceed with a pregnancy based on these test results. The fact that PGD screens embryos in a test tube before implantation, not fetuses already growing in the womb, held tremendous appeal. Allen and I were both pro choice, but we did not want to have an abortion, particularly to avoid having another child like Henry. We were eager to use PGD to ensure a healthy baby.

We also understood that PGD inevitably would result in the creation of embryos that would not be selected for implantation. This was true for almost any couple undergoing in vitro fertilization, where robust, healthy-appearing embryos are implanted, and those that are failing to develop are not. Of course, people who regard embryos as human beings object to creating and discarding embryos in the first place, and are most certainly opposed to IVF and PGD. But IVF is permissible in our society and is pursued by tens of thousands of couples each year. As a result, thousands of embryos are implanted while others are either cryopreserved for future use, donated for medical research, or discarded. Embryos created through our experience with PGD would face a similar fate. While we strongly believe that embryos deserve special respect, as they are cells with the potential to develop into humans once they are implanted into a uterus, we did not view them as people. This mass of undifferentiated cells does not resemble a human being. It cannot reason, and it cannot survive outside of the womb. In contrast, Henry was alive; he could think, feel, smile, and laugh. Also, since we wanted additional children, we would be able to freeze the excess healthy embryos and use them for a future pregnancy.

Testing for HLA—a trait that was critically important to the success of Henry's stem-cell transplant, but not to the survival of the potential child we were testing—was different. Applying PGD in this way was brand-new. It had not yet undergone extensive ethical review or gained the status of moral acceptability. Together with our doctors, we would have to set our own course through this medical frontier.

Years later, when news of the use of PGD for disease prevention and HLA typing first broke, it was often grouped with selection for parental preferences like family balancing to have a child of a specific sex, eye color, sports ability, or IQ and reduced to the politically charged term "designer baby." I had a hard time understanding why anyone would go through the physical pain and expense of PGD solely to produce a daughter to help complete the perfect family (mom, dad, son, daughter), or to have a child who could read by age three (not that it is even possible to test for that). Not all girls want to have tea parties, and even smart kids may not choose to fulfill their academic potential. Any parent who doesn't know that yet will learn it sooner or later. To us, selecting an embryo based on its HLA type did not belong in the same conversation. Our baby's HLA type was not a superficial desire, but a matter of life or death.

Others rightly raised objections to the use of a baby's organs as spare parts. Removing a young child's kidney or liver to aid a sibling is risky, disturbing, ethically questionable, and deserving of serious debate. But using a baby's umbilical cord blood—which was all we were going to do—is different. The blood residing in the umbilical cord, where the stem cells used for bone-marrow transplants are found, are typically thrown away as medical waste after delivery. Retrieving these cells causes no harm to the baby. Essentially, it is lifesaving recycling.

Although Allen and I gave these issues a lot of thought and discussed them at length with our doctors, it was an easy decision to move forward. As with most things in my life, my mom was the first one I called to share our intention to pursue PGD.

I explained the process, and our decision, telling her everything that I had been keeping to myself, and all the reasons that led me to know that this was the exact right thing to do. The procedure would allow us to wrest control of Henry's fate from his defective genetic code. We could have a child whom we would love unconditionally and who would not have Fanconi anemia. We believed that our child would gain satisfaction from the knowledge that he or she had saved a life—a status that is revered in our culture and in the Jewish faith. People have babies for all sorts of reasons, and for us, having a child who could live a long life as well as save another was on the top of the list of good reasons. Leaving matters up to fate fell far short in our minds next to the promise of enlisting with a small group of brilliant and compassionate physicians as pioneers on the forefront of a revolutionary advance in reproductive genetics.

"You know I will support you in whatever you do," my mom explained, predictably, when I finished speaking. "And I know you aren't asking our permission. You never did that much as a child, either," she added, laughing softly. "But I speak for Dad, too, when I say that you have our blessing. We are behind you and will help in any way possible." She hesitated and added, "I totally understand what you are doing because I would have done anything for you."

Though Allen and I would have moved forward regardless of what others said, we greatly appreciated the support of our family and friends—which we received in every single case—because we understood that choosing to pursue PGD would put our family in the crosshairs of what was sure to be a national debate on reproductive health and bioethics. I expected that some people would accuse us of being irresponsible or unethical or even labeling us as murderers, since PGD involved creating and testing embryos, and selecting and implanting only those that met specific criteria. I also knew that there would be strangers—and friends—who would applaud us for being pioneers.

Even if I had known the extent to which I would have to balance feelings and opinions—my own and other people's—I would have proceeded. But I would also have been a lot more apprehensive than I felt at the moment. Instead, primarily I felt relieved—or, more accurately, elated—that there was something we could do to try to save Henry's life. The only way I could live with Henry's prognosis was to do whatever I could to change it, even something that seemed impossible. I knew that if Allen and I could find the right doctors with the right technology—which I believed we had—Henry would survive a previously unsurvivable disease. All of these things created a great and necessary distraction from the unthinkable possibility that he could die.

I couldn't sleep. I was three months pregnant and waiting for the test results that would reveal if the child I was carrying had Fanconi anemia: if both of our children would die before they learned to read, climb a tree, or fall in love. We were expecting a call from Dr. Auerbach later that day. She had received the baby's amniotic fluid and had conducted the test. The results would be revealed that afternoon. I tried to stay upbeat, but I was overcome with dread. I was unwillingly living in a new universe, in which all the things I wanted to care about seemed trivial and stupid. Nothing was as I imagined it would be.

We got lucky.

*D*r. Auerbach called to confirm that the baby I was carrying did not have Fanconi anemia. We also learned that our baby's HLA was as opposite to Henry's as it could possibly be, while retaining the same parents. I cried when I hung up. My tears were still flowing when I called Allen at work to share the great news. I was so overwhelmingly grateful that we were going to have a healthy baby. Before this phone call, and before Dr. Auerbach's news, I had been filled with so much self-doubt. As someone who had wanted to be a mom more than anything else, the idea that I might not have been able to give birth to a healthy child was devastating.

"How are you? How are you feeling?" Allen asked. I could hear the relief and happiness in his voice.

I sat down at the table. I was filled with such enormous relief and excitement: about the new baby, and that we had found PGD, and could save Henry. Allen shared all this with me, of course, and we agreed that I would call our parents to tell them the wonderful news. As I picked up the phone to call my parents, I realized that Fanconi anemia—a disease I had never even heard of before—had, in that one moment nine months earlier, become my filter. Every experience of my life would be affected by the fact that Henry had it. Every ensuing pregnancy would be marred by the fact that the little baby in my belly could have it. Every job that Allen or I considered had to offer medical insurance without preexisting conditions, and with compassion and flexibility. Every relationship had to offer a quiet understanding of our travails, accompanied by the capacity to give without expecting much in return.

In what seemed like a flash, one year passed and on October 25, 1996, Henry celebrated his first birthday. It was a very happy occasion. On the day of his birthday, our family and friends arrived, bearing huge smiles, boxes with bows, and a lot of hope. Henry was a walking Gap ad, wearing tan overalls with a tan-and-blue-striped shirt, flashing that smile that dazzled. He clapped excitedly as each guest arrived and each time he tore the colorful wrapping paper off a new gift. Henry seemed especially happy when his cousin Rachel walked in, decked out in a blue gingham dress with a rounded collar and a big white bow in her hair (already showing signs of the fashion maven she would become). We perched Henry and Rachel on top of our dining-room table, and they proceeded to stick their fingers into the "Happy 1st Birthday Henry and Rachel" cake.

My friends Erica Antonelli and Debbie Blum—each on the verge of marriage and motherhood—stopped by with a present they had made: the front page of a newspaper called *The Henry Tribune* with headlines like: OH HENRY! EVERYONE'S FAVORITE BABY TURNS ONE. BIRTHDAY BOY BANGS ON BONGOS AS WORLD AWAITS CAREER DECISION. And my favorite: MARRIED WITH CHILDREN: DC COUPLE BUCKS TREND.

In addition to Elmo and birthday songs, Allen and I had also chosen to celebrate Henry's first birthday by launching Hope for Henry, a campaign to raise awareness and critical funds for Fanconi anemia research. We knew that saving Henry's life required a battle on two fronts. The first was to find and access the best medical care possible, which we were doing with the help of our doctors and the Fanconi Anemia Research Fund. The second was to raise as much money as we possibly could to fund medical research that would improve bone-marrow-transplant survival rates and reveal a cure.

It was a great day. Henry was healthy and adorable, and surrounded by people he loved. What would turn out to be his very best gift, however, the thing he loved more than anything else, came two months later. Jack Strongin Goldberg arrived on December 28, 1996, in the same hospital where I had been born. He made his entrance at 4:35 in the morning on a warm day after a long labor, near strangulation by his umbilical cord, and an emergency C-section with inadequate anesthesia. The trauma that immediately preceded Jack's birth was erased by the sound of his hearty cry and the fact that he had ten fingers and toes, a healthy heart, and other signs of longed-for newborn normalcy.

A few hours after Jack was born, my mom brought Henry to the hospital to meet his new brother. From outside the plastic bassinet where Jack rested, Henry, age one, leaned in. "Hi Jack," he said, trying out a new word he had learned earlier that day.

That night, as I nursed Jack to sleep, I couldn't stop looking at our new son, whose brown hair and eyes looked like mine, whose dimples came from Allen, and whose perfect health seemed like nothing short of a miracle.

Henry's Favorite Things

- Beanie Babies
- Sleeping in tents
- Making telephone calls
- The polar bears and penguins at the Central Park Zoo
- Knock-knock jokes
- Penny candy
- Soaring down the rock slides on cardboard box tops at Billy Johnson playground in New York City

5

HOPE INTERRUPTED

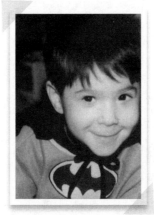

Henry, my hero

$\mathcal{H}$enry met his first hero in the aisles at Sullivan's Toy Store, near our home in downtown Washington. It was among his favorite places to go, especially when in search of something fun. On one particular afternoon, while on his way to the collection of bats, balls, Frisbees, and other flying objects that filled the store's back shelves and our backyard, Henry stopped dead in his tracks.

There he was.

His dark blue cape was spread out as if he were midflight. A mask covered his face, shrouding him in mystery. In the middle of his chest was a big black bat. We didn't even make it out of the store before Henry had freed Batman from his packaging. That night Henry slept with Batman in his clutches.

When it came time for Halloween that year, the black-and-white cow costume was last year's news. Henry was Batman. He was Batman the day after Halloween, and the day after the day after Halloween. He didn't need a holiday to give him permission to honor his hero. Henry quickly accumulated an amazing and diverse collection of Batman action figures that includes, but is not limited to: Code Buster Batman, Future Knight Batman, Gotham Knight Batman, Laser Batman, Power Armor Batman, Rapid Switch Bruce Wayne, Air Attack Batman, Aero Strike Batman, Arctic Batman, Jungle Tracker Batman, Powerwing Batman, Gotham Defender Batman, Photon Armor Batman, Blast Cape Batman, and Fireguard Batman. One time Henry lined all his Batman action figures up head to toe, beginning in our basement. They went all the way up two flights of stairs and into his bedroom, where they wound up in a big pile of awesomeness.

Henry thought it was really cool that Batman protected people from bad guys like Mr. Freeze, the Penguin, and Two-Face, and bad girls like Catwoman, Harley Quinn, and Poison Ivy. He was especially taken with Batman's amazingly equipped utility belt and cool transportation modes like the Batcycle, Batboat, and Batmobile. "Batman is the best Batman is the best Batman is the best," Henry announced to anyone and everyone.

*E*very hero needs a companion. Batman had Robin. The Lone Ranger had Tonto. Shrek had Donkey.

Henry had Jack.

While Jack couldn't help Henry defeat his enemy, Fanconi anemia, he could provide other critical functions expected of a sidekick. When we first brought Jack home from the hospital he was too little, of course, to provide much interaction, but Henry still loved to be near him. Sometimes Henry would tickle Jack's stomach or toes, and other times he would sit right next to him and play with his toys. There was clearly something about Jack that appealed to Henry.

By this time, Henry's heart problems were behind him, his extra thumb had been removed, and his medical care consisted of routine visits to the pediatrician and a few specialists. He handled each appointment as if it was just another part of his routine. He went, got poked with a needle, got a lollipop and a cool Batman Band-Aid, and then went to the park to run and play. At the time, you wouldn't have been able to pick Henry out of a group of kids playing in the park as the child suffering from a fatal disease, although it would be hard to miss the smiling kid in the Batman costume traversing the monkey bars. He most definitely did not think of himself as sick, and neither did we.

My second maternity leave was far less demanding and more peaceful than the first. I'd wake up with Jack, feed him and Henry, and then head out for a walk. It was an unseasonably warm winter that year, and with Jack in the baby carrier, I'd chase fourteen-month-old Henry around the park or play hide-and-seek with him. As Jack slept against my chest, I'd push Henry on the swings. Every month, I looked forward to a night out with the girls, when I'd go meet the Ladies of the Pines for white pizza and eggplant parmesan.

After three months, I returned to work full-time, and we hired a nanny to watch over the boys. Over time, they spent their days running around Guy Mason Playground, chasing each other and any other kid up for joining them. In the evenings, Allen and I would return from work and play with the boys, read to them, listen to music, and blow bubbles for them to pop in the bathtub. We reveled in the normalcy of life with two young children. Allen had just gotten a job with an Internet start-up firm based in Atlanta, so he spent a fair amount of time on the road, a sacrifice we were all willing to make in exchange for the financial return that would allow us to afford the medical care that awaited Henry.

Knowing that Henry's health would not always be as good as it was at this time led us to recognize the importance of living each day to its fullest. We believed that one Halloween costume was never enough and that, with its complement of calcium, ice cream was more than a suitable dinner. Over time we became masters of good living, which would later come in handy when there wasn't much to work with.

But we would do everything we could to delay that day's intrusive arrival.

*F*rom the moment of Henry's diagnosis, Allen and I believed that if we made every call, pulled every string, acted as tireless advocates, and pushed our love and science to their outer limits, Henry would escape his fate. We placed our faith squarely in the promise of PGD.

Recognizing that this option was our best and perhaps only hope to save Henry's life, Allen and I had begun to prepare for our first attempt when I was still pregnant with Jack. We provided blood samples for DNA analysis and HLA typing, met with our doctors, and educated ourselves as best as we could on the process.

PGD begins with IVF, which would make getting pregnant a lot more complicated, painful, and impersonal than my two previous pregnancies. The plan was that when Jack was a few months old, I would begin the IVF process with daily injections of a drug called Lupron to halt my natural egg production. Weeks later, when blood tests confirmed that the Lupron had taken effect, I would add an additional injection of hormones, for a period of six to eleven days, to stimulate superovulation and produce, we hoped, twenty or more eggs, rather than the one egg that I, and most women, typically produce each month. When the eggs reached the appropriate level of maturity, I would take a single injection of human chorionic gonadotropin (hCG) to trigger the final "ripening" of the eggs. Within the next thirty-six hours, before I began to ovulate on my own, my eggs would be retrieved through surgery and united with Allen's sperm. Three days later, one or two cells would be extracted from each fertilized embryo and sent to a lab to determine which embryos were both FA-free and an HLA match. Within two days, the doctors performing the testing would call the doctors in the IVF clinic and tell them which of the embryos to transfer to my uterus. After the procedure, I would take daily injections of progesterone until my pregnancy test. All told, this procedure would take about five weeks. Nine months later, the theory went, we would have a healthy baby— our third child—and be assured that Henry would have the life we meant to give him at birth.

It almost sounded too good to be true.

When we began quietly pursuing PGD in 1996, it was neither on the national news nor featured in fertility clinic advertisements. At that point, it was somewhere between a distant hope and an extraordinary dream shared by a small group of doctors and families who believed in the promise of science.

I had no doubt that if my body would cooperate, our doctors would deliver a baby and give us our boy back. The team we had assembled was comprised of the most brilliant and compassionate doctors, all experts in Fanconi anemia, reproductive health, molecular genetics, or bone-marrow transplantation. Each was a pioneer working at the most controversial edges of science. Each had taken on perplexing medical puzzles that eluded their colleagues and offered hope to patients where otherwise there was none. The challenges they sought placed them before desperate families trying to bring babies into the world or save the ones they had. While success would be a major medical breakthrough, even a miracle, failure would bring death and devastation.

Dr. Arleen Auerbach was, of course, part of the team, and so much more than that. Since we first met her when Henry was just a month old, she had felt familiar enough to be part of our family and has always treated us like we were part of hers. Like our mothers, she was in her sixties, and her children and grandchildren were her life's focus. She spoke directly and authoritatively, and immediately earned our trust and respect. She has provided us with information, access to the world's best doctors, and books for our kids. We supported her research and filled her photo albums and PowerPoint slides with Henry's smiling face. We shared dinners, heartache, and advice on computer software. Dr. Auerbach's office was covered with photos of kids like Henry who were, when it came to science, waiting for something to change. After spending dozens of years confirming death sentences, she saw the potential of PGD to eradicate Fanconi anemia. She encouraged two prominent colleagues of hers—Drs. Hughes and Rosenwaks—to expand the use of PGD beyond testing for the presence of disease by adding HLA typing. She was the one who suggested that they try first with Fanconi anemia, given the dire consequences associated with it. And it was she who identified us as one of only two families that met the stringent criteria that Dr. Hughes set forth for patients selected to serve as PGD pioneers.

Dr. Zev Rosenwaks is the director of the Center for Reproductive

Medicine and Infertility, the world-renowned infertility clinic at New York–Presbyterian Weill Cornell. He is one of the most, if not the most, respected fertility doctors in the world. With leading-man good looks that matched his celebrated reputation, Dr. Rosenwaks emanated confidence, and within minutes of meeting him we had no doubt that we were in the very best hands. He had been part of the team that produced the first test-tube baby, and he had worked on the first PGD case. In 1997, he and Dr. Hughes were able to successfully help a couple—both carriers of the recessive mutation for sickle cell disease—use IVF and PGD to achieve a pregnancy with an unaffected embryo. The couple delivered healthy twins at thirty-nine weeks' gestation and proved that PGD can be a powerful diagnostic tool for carrier couples who want a healthy child and want to avoid the difficult decision of whether to abort an affected fetus. Dr. Rosenwaks's success in helping women get pregnant through IVF has resulted in a celebrity following and a long waiting list.

Once our third baby was born and the umbilical cord blood was retrieved and properly prepared, Dr. John Wagner would perform Henry's stem-cell transplant in Minneapolis. Dr. Wagner is a young, earnest, hard-working, unassuming stem-cell-transplant superstar on the rise. He specializes in Fanconi transplants, which are among the most challenging. He has watched far too many young children die. PGD was the first scientific advancement in a long time that would make his heartbreaking job easier.

As far as we knew, there was not another doctor in the world better equipped and motivated to save Henry's life than Dr. Mark Hughes. In 1993, Dr. Hughes's research was named "one of the ten most significant developments/discoveries in all of science" that year by *Science* magazine. In 1994, he published a paper in the *New England Journal of Medicine* describing the first successful use of PGD for disease prevention. Dr. Hughes, along with colleagues in

London, had used PGD to ensure that a couple at risk of having a child with cystic fibrosis had a healthy baby instead. Dr. Hughes was among the group of nineteen leading bioethicists, sociologists, physicians, scientists, and public-policy professionals recruited by NIH to join the Human Embryo Research Panel, a federal advisory committee charged with creating guidelines for the government's support of embryo research.

Soon thereafter, NIH recruited Dr. Hughes from his lab at Baylor College of Medicine in Houston, Texas. NIH's National Center for Human Genome Research funded Dr. Hughes's work through a government contract with Georgetown University, where he would continue to develop methods for extracting DNA from single cells for genetic diagnosis.

In September 1994, the Human Embryo Research Panel recommended that embryo research be funded by the federal government. The panel found that the "promise of human benefit from research is significant, carrying great potential benefit to infertile couples, families with genetic conditions, and individuals and families in need of effective therapies for a variety of diseases." The NIH Director's Advisory Committee reviewed and approved the panel's report, and President Clinton approved it in December 1994, with the exception of a controversial area of research that involved the creation of human embryos for research. The approved guidelines explicitly supported Dr. Hughes's work on PGD.

Against the recommendations of the medical and bioethics experts on the Human Embryo Research Panel, and to the heartache of families like us, who looked to this science to save our children, in 1995, Congress passed an appropriations bill that overrode the NIH guidelines and completely banned the use of federal funds for research that destroys or seriously endangers human embryos. This provision, known as the Dickey Amendment (after its original author, former Rep. Jay Dickey of Arkansas), seriously hampered Dr. Hughes's work, significantly delayed research advances, and probably ruined a lot of sick children's chances for survival.

The federal ban disallowed Dr. Hughes from performing his work on PGD as part of his position at NIH. It disrupted the work of countless others as well, forcing researchers to seek private funding or to give up their work entirely. Refusing to abandon his research or the families whose lives depended on it, Dr. Hughes had set up a lab as part of an IVF program at Suburban Hospital in Bethesda, Maryland, a private hospital across the street from NIH. There, with private funds, he continued his PGD work, primarily for couples anxious to screen out deadly genetic diseases.

When Allen and I first met Dr. Hughes in the fall of 1996, he made it exceptionally clear that this work was being done on his own time, independent of his work with NIH. The three of us hit it off immediately. He was about a decade older than us, but exuded youthful exuberance and clearly took delight in the possibilities that science could offer couples like us. His eyes sparkled and his smile grew as he looked at the pictures of Henry we had brought with us to the meeting. With each new picture, he paused and really looked at Henry. We thought that once he saw Henry, he couldn't possibly turn us away. We were right.

Over lunch in Georgetown, he told us what to expect, assessed the potential for success and failure, and discussed the ethical implications. From the moment we met Dr. Hughes, his passion for science and his sense of ethical responsibility has been transparent and admirable. He spent more time talking with us about the risks associated with being among the first to try PGD than he did on its promise. It was he who would later personally meet Allen for the handoff of the cells for testing or call to deliver our test results, as difficult as those calls were, or to check in on Henry. He didn't look at saving Henry as a means to career advancement, although it certainly would be, but as his responsibility. To him, Henry was the little boy in the picture who deserved a chance to live, taped to the wall in his lab for all to see. WE CAN SAVE HIS LIFE, read the note posted near the picture. Our frequent late-night e-mail exchanges were proof that he wouldn't rest until he figured out how to save our son.

Over time, like us, I think that each of these doctors, as they got to know Henry, came to believe that he was invincible. For that to be true, each of them had to excel at his or her area of expertise and then hand us off to the next physician in the chain. These pioneers, and this precarious set of links, would determine the course of Henry's life.

On January 9, 1997, when Jack was just thirteen days old, I sat on the couch in the floral nursing nightgown and matching bathrobe that Allen's parents recently had given me. I heard a thud on our front porch and got up to get the newspaper. It was dark and cold outside. Inside, it was warm and filled with joy. Jack was healthy and thriving. We were about to start PGD. Everything was good. I returned to the couch, picked up my mug of coffee, and began to read *The Washington Post*.

Several pages into the front section, all that was good in my life was quickly forgotten. In bold letters over an article in the front section, I read that Dr. Mark Hughes, our savior, was being accused of violating the federal ban on embryo research with his work on PGD, in violation of the Dickey Amendment. Shocked into high alert, I sat upright and continued to read. My stomach progressively tied up in knots and it got harder to breathe. I could not believe what I was reading. It did not make any sense. Although Dr. Hughes did not conduct any embryo research at NIH, he was charged with violating the congressional ban because his PGD work at nearby Suburban Hospital—where he was already working on our case—employed

NIH research fellows and scientific equipment, like *a refrigerator*, that NIH said had been moved to Suburban without NIH approval. While I read the words on the page, the only thing I could see written in black and white before me was one sentence.

Henry is going to die.

According to NIH sources cited in a *Chicago Tribune* article that same day, Dr. Hughes got into trouble because one of the four research fellows assigned to assist him, all of whom were funded by NIH, was worried that experiments they were conducting violated federal law. Apparently, the fellow reported his concern to Genome Center officials, who ordered the investigation that resulted in Dr. Hughes's termination. I'm neither a policy expert nor am I supportive of the federal ban on embryo research, so it seemed simply absurd that a refrigerator and one research fellow separated a brilliant doctor from the only chance my son had to live past age five. Dr. Hughes's work wasn't violating any law; it was saving Henry's life. My rage was all-consuming. There I was with my newborn, my coffee, and my newspaper, filled with a fury I had never experienced before. I had no one to yell at, no one to strike. I looked over at Jack, peacefully unaware of his mother's anguish, and sobbed.

Each new story further demonizing Dr. Hughes in the *Post* and other newspapers delivered a new rush of terror and shock and rage. Together they threatened to slap the joy out of my life and steal my dream of Henry's survival.

Initially, Georgetown University released supportive statements, but the reality was that Dr. Hughes's work did not comport with the Jesuit institution's religious ban on embryo research. Within days, Dr. Hughes resigned from his position rather than agree to terminate his research. But without a job and access to the equipment he needed, he was denied the ability to continue the research upon which Henry's life depended.

All the optimism and promise fueled by that first phone call from Dr. Auerbach was gone in a flash. We were desperate and scared. We had diapers to change, children to nourish, and a lot of living to do, as one-fifth of Henry's predicted life span had already passed us by and we wanted so badly to live each day to its fullest, for happiness to win over fear. Allen and I immediately called Dr. Hughes to offer support, but there was only so much we could do, except suffer from the sidelines. Not only did Dr. Hughes have to leave his lab at Suburban Hospital, where he had been preparing for our case, he also faced congressional hearings that vilified him and threatened his career and our prospects. Six months later, as I anxiously read the testimony that Dr. Harold Varmus, director of the NIH, delivered before the investigating Senate committee, I wondered how it could be possible that Dr. Varmus and his staff didn't know or approve of Dr. Hughes's work on PGD, given that he had been recruited in part based on this very area of expertise.

More months passed, we waited, and Henry's blood counts fell. Without a perfectly matched sibling donor, his transplant survival rates remained dismally low, and we did our best to cling to hope, which was more challenging with each passing day. We stayed in close contact with Dr. Hughes, Dr. Auerbach, and other members of our growing medical team in search of alternatives. Because no other doctor in the country was engaged in this groundbreaking PGD research, there was no one else to turn to. Shy of rolling the dice and getting pregnant again on our own, which had only an 18.75 percent chance of producing an HLA-matched sibling, there was nothing to do but wait.

Throughout 1997, Allen was unwavering in his belief that Dr. Hughes would soon find a suitable home for his work and would resume his efforts to help us save Henry's life. The two kept in frequent touch via e-mail. Those correspondences, paired with Allen's patience and focus on the endgame—specifically, Dr. Hughes's securing a new position absent the government's stranglehold, where he would finally be free to conduct his breakthrough research—provided Allen with all the encouragement he needed. I had moments of confidence, but far less often. Although I knew that Dr. Hughes was committed to his work and to us, I was also scared and in need of concrete evidence that things were progressing in our favor. With the passing of months and the continuing decline of Henry's blood counts, I had an increasingly difficult time taking solace in Allen's optimism. Without his saying it, I think Allen grew tired of my need to rehash, yet again, my mounting concern and need for additional encouragement from Dr. Hughes. Perhaps my anxiety threatened to weaken his resolve. Maybe I was just asking the wrong questions.

"Aren't you worried that by the time Dr. Hughes finds a job, it will be too late to help Henry?" I would query nervously from my side of the bed in our darkened room at night.

"No," Allen would reply.

And with that, the conversation would end. Over time and with practice, I learned that a better conversation starter was "I'm feeling really anxious about the amount of time Dr. Hughes is taking to get settled into a new job. How are you feeling?"

"Just look at him," he'd say, gazing adoringly at Henry, who was building and knocking down huge block towers in our family room. "We have the best doctors and the greatest love on our side. It is all going to work out. Just not exactly on our timetable."

Simply relating the content of these conversations denies the nuance that better characterized Allen's and my perspectives and their effect on our relationship. I am neither a cynic nor a worrier; Allen isn't a Pollyanna, nor is he shallow. Allen and I didn't fight, nor did we live in silence. Our mutual aversion to conflict and our greatest common goal guided our focus toward what was good and right in our relationship—our shared values and interests, and especially our endless love for our children.

There were times, however, that I felt so damn lonely. When Henry and Jack were babies, few of our friends had children, and of those who did, none had anything approaching the issues we faced. Prior to Henry's birth, I'd been very lucky in that things had mostly gone my way, so I had very little experience in allowing myself to be vulnerable and asking for help. Although our family and friends were clear about their desire to hold our hands all the way, no matter what, it was hard for me to be open and honest with them about the pain and fear I felt. It's not that I didn't talk to people. During those times, I was awfully grateful that I had friends like the Ladies of the Pines and Karen Chaikin, Debbie, Val, and Susie Weiner, who never seemed to tire of me. Karen lived in Cleveland and we logged in many hours on the telephone, talking from our respective couches, hundreds of miles apart. However, I never shared everything I truly felt; I couldn't bear to hear the words come out of my own mouth.

Though my parents and I have always been extremely close, I couldn't even be fully honest and open with them. Part of it may have been a reluctance to cause them additional pain by letting them know how much I was suffering. Part of it may have been that I couldn't bear to hear how bad this experience was for them. Maybe I just didn't want the responsibility for helping them feel better. I had very little left to give, even to them.

Although I was, and remain, resistant to joining a group whose central bond is a shared illness, I really wanted, even needed, to befriend another mother in my shoes. And so when the Fanconi Anemia Research Fund invited our family to Camp Sunshine, where more than sixty FA families meet once a year to learn from doctors and one another, Allen and I agreed that we would go. Allen's main goal was to meet the doctors we had yet to meet and get more information on FA. My main goal was to find a friend.

In May 1997, we packed up the kids and drove to Maine. It took us nearly ten hours to get to Portland, where we spent a beautiful afternoon at Old Orchard Beach with my college roommate Jane Esselstyn; and another six to get up the nerve to leave Portland and drive the last thirty miles to Camp Sunshine in Casco, Maine.

The day we arrived, I met my friend. Her name was Lisa Nash, and she was the only other person in the world who could possibly understand what I was going through. She was the mother of the other family identified by Dr. Auerbach as fitting Dr. Hughes's strict criteria—and she, too, was waiting for him. Like us, they had been asked not to talk with other families about PGD because it was un-proven and unavailable to others who would undoubtedly crave its promise, but we could certainly talk with each other. And we did. Many, many times.

As I came to learn, Lisa and her husband, Jack Nash, had a daughter named Molly who was one year older than Henry. They lived in Denver, Colorado, and had traveled even farther to get to the gathering in Maine, desperate to learn more about the availabil-ity of PGD—and other alternatives, should Dr. Hughes be unable to help them. Like us, they got a call from Dr. Auerbach more than one year earlier, but unlike us, they were not pregnant at the time. Therefore, they started to pursue PGD right away. They were in the middle of their first PGD attempt when the news about Dr. Hughes and the potential violation of the embryo research ban broke. As it happened, and for reasons that go well beyond my understanding of molecular genetics, their DNA sequencing was difficult to diagnose. That complicated their case and led Dr. Hughes eventually to work on our case first, after which he would focus on saving Molly. Given the uncertainties that existed and the concentration required by the research, it was easier for Dr. Hughes to focus on just one family at a time. I can only imagine how difficult it was for the Nashes to have had the opportunity to try PGD, only to have it interrupted by poli-tics, genetics, and other things beyond their control.

Despite the assault, Dr. Hughes refused to allow politics to destroy the science, and seven months after the *Post* article, he found a home at a private lab at Wayne State University in Michigan, where he could continue his research. Unfortunately, all the preliminary work Dr. Hughes had done—our DNA and HLA typing, as well as our gene sequencing—was gone, as he'd been unable to take his research with him when he lost his job.

That fall, while Drs. Hughes and Rosenwaks got ready for us, Henry turned two. The day was sunny and bright, mirroring our spirits. Perched in his chair at our dining-room table, with light streaming through the windows, wearing overalls and a Batman party hat, Henry ate the cake I had made. His chocolate-covered dimples threatened to melt my heart. He squealed with delight as Allen suspended him by his ankles and repeatedly dunked him through the net on the Playskool basketball hoop we got him. "More, more, more!" he yelled whenever he sensed Allen tiring of the game. My parents gave Henry a brand-new red-blue-and-green tricycle. He immediately jumped on the bike and started riding it across our small living room, into the dining room and kitchen, turning the area into a race track. "Look me! Look me!" he exclaimed as he breezed by.

$\mathcal{F}$inally, two months later, in December 1997, while on a family vacation in Florida, Allen gave me my first shot of Lupron, signaling the start of our experiment with PGD and our battle to save Henry's life. Everything was in place: Our doctors had the technology and the team ready to successfully execute the procedure, and our families had offered to provide the financial support that the insurance company had flatly refused. Despite being weary from the fight, Allen and I were more than ready to see where the power of our love combined with the possibilities of science could take us.

By this time, Henry's blood tests showed that his health was beginning to fail. His platelets—the blood cells necessary for clotting—were at 71,000, far below the normal count of 150,000 to 400,000. His absolute neutrophil count, an indicator of his ability to fight infection, was at 800, far below the desired level of 5,000. Henry's diminishing blood counts didn't negatively affect his day-to-day wellbeing, but they served as a worrisome reminder that we were in a race against time.

Therefore, when the time came two and a half weeks later to relocate for several weeks to Weill Cornell Center for Reproductive Medicine and Infertility in New York City to begin our first IVF cycle, we were more than ready to leave our home, jobs, school, and friends in Washington. Both of our employers gave us permission to work remotely from our hotel in New York. I was so excited about what we were going to do that I wanted to tell the lady in the newspaper circulation department why I was putting my paper on hold with no restart date, but I stuck to the facts. We left our pet fish with my sister Abby and picked up the maternity clothes I had lent her, sure that I'd need them soon enough. We packed a tent for the kids to sleep in at our hotel and filled their heads with exciting stories about adventures to museums, carousels, and the Batman store (known to others as the Warner Bros. store). At one and two years old, they were too young to understand the purpose of our trip to Gotham City, so we didn't try to explain.

Henry's Favorite Things

- Having lemonade stands
- Shabbat Sing at Gan Hayeled Preschool
- *Lady and the Tramp* I and II
- Wearing a tuxedo
- Slow dancing
- Chocolate croissants
- Harry Potter, "The boy who lived"

TAKE ONE

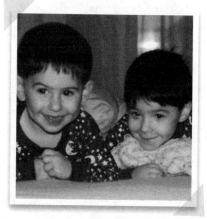

Jack and Henry, the Dynamic Duo, prepare for bedtime

On January 4, 1998, we drove to New York City. No one we passed on Route 95 north that day, walked by on the streets of New York, or sat next to in the fertility clinic knew anything of our challenges. But I had a newfound sense of importance and focus. My feeling of privilege and honor that we could be the first to benefit from a technology that was sure to save countless lives in the future overshadowed my trepidation about being a research subject for the first time in my life and entering a foreign medical world that would strip away any privacy surrounding the creation of our next baby.

We made arrangements to stay at the Helmsley Medical Tower Apartments, just upstairs from Cornell's IVF clinic, for the remaining weeks that it would take to complete the process and return home pregnant. That first morning, I set two alarm clocks for 7:00 a.m.; neither was necessary. I walked excitedly into the IVF clinic, where I wrote three checks totaling more than $10,000. I also submitted signed consent forms for the IVF procedure, the embryo transfer, the study of nonviable preembryos, and the cryopreservation—or freezing for future use—of embryos unused in our IVF cycle. For us, that last form held incredible promise, as our unused embryos could serve two important purposes: We could use Fanconi-free embryos in the future to have another guaranteed-healthy baby; and diseased embryos could unlock the mysteries of Fanconi and with that, reveal a cure.

I sat alone in a chair in the far corner. An hour or so later, as I lay cold and naked but for an ill-fitting hospital gown on an examining table in the midst of a transvaginal ultrasound, the sonographer muttered something about a dominant follicle. She then finished what she was doing and sent me on my way. I had no idea what she was looking for, what she had found, or what "dominant follicle" meant, but it was over so quickly I didn't have time to ask. I didn't know anyone else who had ever done IVF, so I didn't have anyone to call. I took the elevator downstairs, walked to the coffee shop next to the hotel, and grabbed some milk and doughnuts for the kids' breakfast. When I got to the room, Allen and the boys were just waking up. The kids ate inside their tent in our hotel room

"How'd it go?" Allen asked, handing me a hot cup of coffee.

"I have no idea," I said.

The kids crawled out from the tent, and the conversation turned to our upcoming adventure in Central Park. After breakfast, Allen, Henry, Jack, and I walked to the Central Park Zoo to visit the polar bears and penguins, and to feed and pet the llamas and sheep. This was the first of many trips to Central Park to visit the zoo, ride the carousel, careen down the rock slide on pieces of cardboard at the Billy Johnson Playground on East Sixty-seventh Street, or watch street performers, one of whom told Henry the funniest knock-knock joke any of us have ever heard to this day. As we walked through Central Park, a performer approached Henry.

"Knock, knock!" he said.

"Who's there?" Henry said, all smiles.

"Cowp," said the performer. Henry was confused. He had heard plenty of knock-knock jokes, but this was a new one.

"Cowp who?" asked Henry. The performer laughed, and Henry looked confused. Henry repeated, "Cowp who?"

"Cow poo. You said cow poo." Henry, realizing it at the same time, burst into a fit of giggles.

As promised, later that afternoon, one of the nurses called me with my daily instructions. She abruptly told me that I would have to remain on the Lupron for four additional days, after which I should return to the clinic for further testing. Apparently, I had begun to ovulate on my own, which is not what we wanted. The Lupron was meant to prevent my body from going through its normal monthly cycle, so that the hormone shots that would follow the Lupron injections could produce more eggs than normal. The doctors wanted to see if a little more time would enable the drug to be more effective in shutting down my body's natural cycle of ovulation. Before I could react or even begin to ask the questions that were flying through my head, the phone call was over.

Just as when Henry was born, I racked my brain to see if I had done anything wrong. I had followed the instructions and done everything they had told me to do. I was trying so hard to be the very best mom I could be. After all we had been through, it seemed only fair that things should go smoothly. You'd think that I would have dropped the whole "fair" thing by this point, but it was hard to shed my faith and optimism. I was disappointed, but determined. Allen retained his focus on the endgame and took the delay in stride.

"We always said we wanted to live in New York," he said. "Now we have a little more time to do the things we love to do here." Of course, it was worth the wait, but it was also costly, as Allen and I would have to pay more than $1,000 for the four additional hotel nights, even at the hospital's discount rate. This was the Upper East Side of Manhattan, after all. The financial costs associated with this extra week in New York exceeded the monthly mortgage payment for our small row house in Washington.

That night, I got the flu. Henry caught it the next day. And then Jack. Allen spent the days filling prescriptions; taking Henry and Jack to the hospital in Hackensack, New Jersey, where Henry's hematologist, Dr. Al Gillio, was based; and taking care of all of us. My friends Karen and Susie, former residents of New York City, had soup and a chicken delivered to our hotel room. My parents drove from Washington to New York to help us out.

"Don't worry, Hank!" my dad said when he entered and saw Henry lying on the hotel bed, his face flushed with fever. "You're going to be shipshape in no time."

We spent sleepless nights taking baths with the kids to try to get their fevers down.

Despite the sore throat, hot sweats, and chills, each afternoon I would inject my dose of Lupron and hope like hell it was doing what it needed to do.

Twenty-four days and an equal number of Lupron injections later, after a week in and out of the IVF clinic in New York, Allen and I learned that despite all the love and hope and medical intervention, our attempt was a bust. That night I was instructed to take an injection of a drug called hCG—not to release the twenty-plus eggs we were striving for but the one, unwanted egg that my body had created on its own, which was interfering with the PGD cycle and would never be fertilized and never produce our dream child. I dug my hands into the brown paper bag filled with all of my syringes, needles, and medication and found the unopened bottle of hCG. Allen and I stepped into the cluttered, off-white, undecorated hotel-room bathroom. Wet towels from our many baths had soaked the floor. I kicked them to the side and pulled my pajama pants down. My legs were covered with bruises. With my right hand, I felt for the spot that the nurse had described by phone as the destination for my shot. Allen counted down, three-two-one, and penetrated my skin with the thick needle. The medication burned as it flowed into my bloodstream. I leaned over the sink, sobbing. My head was throbbing and my stomach was bloated from all the medication, my thighs and hips were bruised from injections, and my heart was shattered.

That week, Henry's platelets fell to 31,000—their lowest level ever.

Henry's Favorite Things

- Ari, Jake, and Simon
- Playing Uno, Skip Bo, and Blink
- His teachers Elaine, Big D, and Little L
- Tortilla chips with lots of salt at Cactus Cantina
- Counting by 5s
- Party favors
- Foreign currency

7

HOPE FOR HENRY

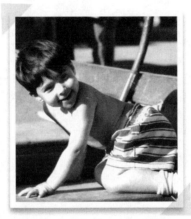

Henry playing in Laguardia, Spain

$\mathcal{I}$t never occurred to me that there were many desperate couples who tried IVF, only to see it fail, before Louise Brown, the first test-tube baby, was born. But as Allen, Henry, Jack, and I drove home from New York City that January, I felt naïve for thinking that PGD would work the first time, and stupid for asking my sister to return my maternity clothes. This medical breakthrough would require more perseverance, time, and money than we had anticipated.

I was painfully conscious of the fact that the first time, the failure belonged to me. My body had failed me; and I had failed Henry, Jack, Allen, and our doctors. The second time around, I would make it right.

Although we had no doubt that our team of doctors was doing everything humanly possible to help us save Henry, we also were preparing for plan B. Just in case. Over the years, with the help of family and friends, we organized bone-marrow drives from Washington to St. Louis in hopes of finding a backup donor, should our dream of PGD go unanswered. We also raised more than $150,000 for the Fanconi Anemia Research Fund to improve bone-marrow-transplant recovery rates and other treatments for FA. Although the prospects of this backup plan were bleak, it provided us with some hope and the ability to try to help others in the same predicament who may not have access to the resources we had. Importantly, all the hard work provided a much-needed distraction from my increasing fear in the face of Henry's steadily declining blood counts.

Two weeks after returning home from our initial defeat, we tried PGD again. I boarded the Amtrak train in Washington and headed alone to New York City. With me, I brought high hopes and another round of checks totaling just over $10,000 to cover the cost of my treatment. I also brought a laptop computer that would enable me to keep working for my employer, Neighborhood Reinvestment, so I could continue my satisfying job of helping people buy and maintain homes. I also needed to preserve my income and, even more important, health insurance for my family. Because Allen worked for an Internet start-up company whose benefits were less comprehensive, our family depended on the insurance provided through my job. As the train headed north, I longed for someone to talk to or something to read that would help me understand what to expect with PGD or, better yet, some success rates that would encourage me that this time things would be different. Instead I read *Us Weekly* and *Vogue*, and learned what not to wear.

"No dominant follicles," declared the sonographer early the next morning. A month earlier, those three words would have meant nothing to me. Today, they meant that the Lupron worked, I was not ovulating, and my body was poised to save Henry's life. The nurse took a blood sample to test my estrogen level for confirmation. All I had to do was wait seven or so hours until the IVF nurse called to let me know that I could start the next phase of treatment. To tell me that this time, everything would be different.

I took the elevator down to the street level, opened the door to the freezing cold outside, and began to walk. I didn't have any particular destination, just a need to pass the time until the call. For many long, quiet hours, I followed the green traffic lights wherever they took me. I walked slowly, getting lost in the crowd pushing their way across Park Avenue. Sometimes I would make it to Central Park, where I could walk for hours undisturbed. I didn't care where I went; I just needed to keep walking, to keep hoping.

I eventually took the train to my Aunt Alice and Uncle Peter's house in Morristown, New Jersey. I was resting on the couch, fighting off a blinding, Lupron-induced headache, when Dr. Rosenwaks called. The news wasn't good. He told me that I needed to remain on the Lupron for four more days, at which point I should return for further testing. Despite the two months on Lupron, my estrogen level was still twice as high as it needed to be to safely begin taking the Follistim, the drug to stimulate my egg production. I hung up the phone and cried. We had already waited so long to get to this point. As I sat on the couch hiding under a blanket, I wondered what I was doing there. I should be home with the boys, enjoying what little time I had with Henry. What was I doing spending the days walking the streets of New York, waiting on disappointing test results? But of course, going home was out of the question. Giving up meant that Henry would die, and there was no way I was going to sit back and let that happen.

I pulled myself together and called Allen at home. He was in the middle of giving the boys a bath. I could hear them laughing in the background. He could hear the disappointment lingering at the edge of my voice. But being nearly two hundred miles away, there wasn't much he could do to make me feel better.

"I know it's hard," he said. "But we have time to keep going."

"I know," I said. "I just wish I could be there with you guys. I want to be blowing bubbles and watching the boys catch them on their noses."

"We'll be there in a couple of days and we'll have a great week-end," he said. "Try to focus on the big picture; it's just a few extra days. It's so worth it."

"You're right. I just wish I could read them a story tonight."

We said good night and a little while later, the phone rang again.

"Mommy," Henry said. "Will you read a story?"

"I would love to, sweetie. Which one should we read?"

"*Goodnight Moon.*"

And so, with Jack and Henry tucked under their covers in Washington, and me tucked under mine in Morristown, I "read" my babies a story, which by that point I knew by heart, and kissed them all good night.

Allen later told me that after we hung up, he and Henry had cuddled inside the fort they had made of sheets on Henry's bed. They spoke in hushed tones so they wouldn't wake up Jack, asleep in the next room. Their headlamps, a camping mainstay that had become standard equipment in our house, lit their way. "Dad, I want to see Mom," Henry said.

"Hen, I told you that she needs to stay in New York a little longer, but you, me, and Jack are gonna head up this weekend to see her."

"When?"

"In less than forty-eight hours."

"That's too big. Tomorrow?"

"How about in two days? Does that sound better?"

"Yeah!"

*W*hile I waited for Allen and the boys to arrive, and to return to the IVF clinic later that week, I turned my attention to work and spending time with friends in New York City. I went window shopping with my college friend Susie, who drove in from Connecticut, and ate delicious Italian desserts at one of John Lennon's old haunts, Café La Fortuna in Manhattan's Upper West Side, with my elementary-school buddy Rich Freedman.

I also decided to chronicle my experience with PGD so that no other family would have to go into this as blindly as we had. Although each family would inevitably experience PGD differently, facing a variety of outcomes and decisions along the way, at least I could provide insights as to what to expect practically, physically, and emotionally. There is a significant amount of literature on what to expect while undergoing IVF, but PGD is different because you are enduring the procedure at the same time that your child is slowly dying. This race against time makes the inevitable delays and disappointments nearly unbearable.

I also recognized that this medical breakthrough—whenever it happened—would result in an extraordinary amount of media coverage, and would spark ethics and policy debates. I knew that it would be easier for people to oppose abstractions, like designer babies and embryonic stem-cell research, than it would be to challenge medical advances that could save a child like Henry. So in return for my gift of being able to be among the first, I carefully chronicled each injection. I kept track of every egg I produced, every embryo that was successfully fertilized, and every disappointing test result. In my journal, I described the heights of my hope and the depths of my despair.

On the day of my appointment, I left my aunt and uncle's house in Morristown at five forty-five a.m., and drove their car into New York City for further testing. I gave a few vials of blood, had a sonogram, and was back in the car heading to New Jersey three hours later. I spent the day napping, working, and wishing I were with Allen, Henry, and Jack. That evening, I learned that despite forty-two shots of Lupron, my estrogen was still too high to safely begin IVF. On the phone, Dr. Rosenwaks presented three possible courses of action. I could immediately begin taking Follistim, a medicine that stimulates the production of multiple eggs, and come in for careful daily monitoring since I would be considered high-risk because of the possibility of hyperstimulating my ovaries. Or I could increase the number of daily Lupron shots to two a day for a few days and then start Follistim. Or I could take a shot of hCG like the last time, go back home, and wait a few weeks to begin the process all over again.

I simply couldn't board the train back home defeated yet again. I also couldn't bear the thought of remaining in this holding pattern for another few days while I sat waiting too far away from Allen and the boys. I could not wait any longer. After some pleading on my part and much consideration on his, Dr. Rosenwaks agreed to pursue the first option: Immediately begin the Follistim and proceed with caution. That night I lined up all the needles and vials of Lupron, Follistim, and the diluent to mix it in. I read and reread the directions, mixed the medication precisely, and carefully injected the Lupron and then the Follistim into my sore thighs, bruised from months of Lupron injections. The medication burned as I injected it, but I didn't care. It felt so good to have forward momentum. Over the next week or two, Dr. Rosenwaks's job was to achieve a balance between giving me enough Follistim to produce a considerable number of eggs (hopefully ten or more) without hyperstimulating me (associated with risks including nausea, difficulty breathing, and blood clotting, among others) and having to cancel the whole cycle. His sterling reputation is based on his expertise in these matters.

My last real study of genetics was in preparation for my sixth-grade science-fair project on Gregor Mendel. Despite my taking home first place, I was hardly an expert at age twelve, let alone now, at age thirty-two; but I understood that each fertilized egg had a 25 percent chance of having FA. Because the chance of any one being both healthy *and* an HLA match was merely 18.75 percent, the more eggs we tested, the greater the likelihood that we would beat these daunting odds. Although I hoped for twenty eggs, at this point I was so desperate that I would have settled for anything more than the one I could produce each month on my own.

The next day, Allen, Henry, and Jack finally arrived in New York City, where we spent a long weekend at the Helmsley Medical Tower Apartments for yet another $1,000. I waited for them in the lobby, and when I saw Allen pushing the double stroller through the large glass doors, I thought my heart would explode from excitement. Henry jumped out of his seat and ran into my arms. It had been six days since I'd seen him, but the way he held on to me, you would have thought we'd been apart for years.

Like he usually did, Jack followed his big brother's lead and, though a little more slowly and clumsily, he also ran out of the stroller and grabbed on to me. Henry made room, allowing Jack space in my arms. Although brotherhood is often fraught with competition, Henry and Jack's relationship seemed to escape that. Instead of viewing Jack as an adversary or worse, as an object of envy given his clean bill of health, Henry saw Jack as a best friend and, as such, someone to look out for. Their closeness was a source of joy for Allen and me.

After dropping off their bags and bundling up, we headed straight for Central Park. It was a crisp and sunny February day. Allen and I each grabbed a stroller handle, and we walked together to the carousel. The music was festive, the lights were bright, and the boys were happy. Henry climbed up onto the black panther, and we boosted Jack onto a white horse. The carousel began to spin. I was dizzy and happy. It felt great to be together again, absent the burden of fear and loneliness weighing me down in the preceding days.

From the hotel, I had easy access to the IVF clinic several floors below, and Henry could be admitted to New York–Presbyterian Hospital Well Cornell for an endocrine workup. He needed to be tested for a growth hormone deficiency; to undergo a hearing and vision screening; to have kidney scans; and he had to visit a neurologist, as well. Fanconi anemia can wreak havoc on all these systems. Henry was just over two at the time, and although he was developing normally, his doctors wanted to rule out any further complications. With each result, I held my breath. In every case, the news was good.

Henry's tests required an overnight stay, so Allen and Henry slept in the hospital while Jack and I returned to the hotel several blocks away so I could go to my early morning appointment. These separations were difficult because those were the times Allen and I most needed to be together for emotional support.

First thing the next morning, I took Jack with me to the IVF clinic for my daily blood work and sonogram, and then we were to meet up with Henry and Allen. When we arrived at the hospital, Dr. Auerbach was already there. She told us that Dr. Hughes had a family emergency. His wife, Claudia, had been found to be ill with cancer after a long remission. We had grown very close with Dr. Hughes, and he and Allen had developed a particularly strong bond. He was such a wonderful, supportive advocate, doctor, and friend to us. Our hearts broke for him, and for ourselves.

Despite his own challenges, Dr. Hughes assured us that he would oversee our testing. That day, we learned the good news that Henry's platelets had increased to 47,000—the highest they had been in months. Though they were still far below normal, they were well above the level of 10,000 that would necessitate a platelet transfusion and signal that we had run out of time. My ovaries were getting big and, succumbing to my desperation for encouragement, the doctors at Cornell predicted that I had ten or more eggs on each side. That night, the four of us went to my aunt and uncle's house in Morristown, New Jersey, where we would stay until my egg retrieval.

Each day that February, I got up at five forty-five a.m., kissed my still-sleeping husband and children, and began the two-and-a-half-hour roundtrip drive into the city for a quick blood test and sonogram. Although I would return exhausted, I wanted nothing more than to spend my time with Allen and the kids. We took advantage of the snow on the ground and made snowmen. "I'll make one of you if you make one of me," Henry said. In the end, we made a family of four—Mommy, Daddy, Henry, and Jack, each adorned with grapes for eyes, a carrot nose, raisins for the mouth, and our hats and gloves, which made them cute, and us cold. Afterward, we warmed up over hot chocolate and movies.

We discovered local parks, wandered around Short Hills Mall, and played with Batman toys. Each evening the nurse called to give me my drug dosages. I took my injections, read stories to the boys, and fell asleep, only to start the cycle again. Nearly two weeks after arriving in New York, I was instructed to take hCG, this time to release the twenty or more eggs in my overfilled ovaries. As Allen injected the shot—a nearly two-inch needle into my skin (this was no allergy shot or tetanus booster)—I felt prouder of myself and my body than I had been years earlier, when I was much more athletic, following a hundred-mile bike ride or a twenty-mile run. With the help of our doctors, I believed that my body would do the impossible and remove the word "fatal" from Henry's disease.

*T*wo days later, I had surgery to remove the twenty-four eggs I had produced, which were immediately united with Allen's sperm in a miracle of science. That was the first time I met my nurse Ruby, a soft-spoken, kind woman. She held my hand in hers and comforted me with her smooth, deep West Indian–accented voice as I was wheeled into the operating room, and again when I awoke from anesthesia. It was as if she understood what was at stake and was personally invested in being there by my side as we intervened to twist Henry's fate. That night Allen drove Henry and Jack home to Washington so I could rest and prepare for the next phase. As I did most nights throughout this cycle, I called Lisa Nash to tell her how we were progressing, both of us aware that it wasn't only Henry's life that was at stake.

The next day, we learned that eighteen eggs had successfully fertilized. If the statistics proved correct, we should get four or five Fanconi-free, perfect HLA matches—one or more of which could be Henry's savior and (because our success would make it the Nashes' turn), in a way, Molly Nash's as well.

As I lay resting, overwhelmed at our good fortune, Dr. Hughes called from his office in Detroit to remind me of all the challenges we could face over the next few days, during which doctors at Cornell hospital would perform the embryo biopsies and Dr. Hughes and his lab staff would conduct the genetic testing. I wanted to cover my ears—the way Jack did when Henry was saying something he didn't like—and bask in possibility, but Dr. Hughes was committed to ensuring that we were always well informed, so that we could make the best, most educated decisions. He carefully explained this war of attrition. Some of the embryos would not grow in the petri dish past the two-to-three-cell stage and therefore would neither be tested nor be able to produce a pregnancy. Others would not survive the cell biopsy required for the genetic testing. Then it was possible that the equipment might fail to deliver any results at all. Even if the equipment functioned properly, the results might not be definitive, meaning that the particular extracted cell might not give us the information about FA or HLA type that we so desperately needed.

Dr. Hughes was straightforward and prepared to talk until I was satisfied that I knew everything there was to know at this stage, which truthfully was more than I wanted to hear. Some of the issues Dr. Hughes raised are realities of IVF and PGD. Some embryos are simply not strong enough to survive even the natural process resulting in miscarriage, and others can't withstand medical intervention. But much of what we discussed was simply part of life on the front lines of a medical breakthrough.

Despite all the preparation, the equipment and protocol had not yet been tested on a real case like ours. I called Allen to share my conversation with Dr. Hughes. Allen listened and then asked me if I had asked whether, if we had multiple healthy HLA matches, we could implant at least one female embryo. Of course, I hadn't. His steadfast faith in our doctors and the promise of science blinded him to the fact that we were on the medical frontier. Despite everything we had already endured, he still thought it would be easy, and was already thinking about the gender of our new baby. I hoped that he was right, but I did not share his confidence.

I spent a day alone in New Jersey, waiting for Allen to return, trying not to overworry about the possibilities of failure. Thankfully, my job was demanding, and I had plenty of work to keep me occupied. The next day, Allen returned to New York and we went to Cornell hospital to speak with the embryologist, Dr. Kangpu Xu. We learned that he had successfully extracted two cells each from fourteen embryos, giving Dr. Hughes the opportunity to run two simultaneous tests on each embryo to increase his certainty with the results. There were still four embryos from which he had yet to extract cells for testing. We returned one hour later to learn that he had removed one cell each from two; the other two had ceased to grow.

Allen took the vials of thirty cells from sixteen embryos, which had been meticulously labeled, carefully packed in ice, and stored in a Styrofoam box. We walked out to the intersection of Seventieth Street and York Avenue and hailed a cab to take Allen to the airport, where he would board a plane and fly to Detroit. Dr. Hughes would be waiting, to take the cells to the lab without delay.

"Thank you so much for doing this for me," I said to Allen. It had been my idea that he personally carry the cells on the flight to Detroit, despite his insistence—along with Dr. Hughes's—that we could put the box on the plane and it would arrive safely. I didn't believe that there was a pilot or flight attendant who could possibly appreciate the value of the contents in that bland white package in the way that Allen did. There was no way I was letting those cells out of our hands for even a minute. A cab pulled over. Afraid to put the box down, we didn't even dare hug. I quickly kissed Allen. "I love you," I whispered, as I stood alone on the sidewalk, watching the cab get lost in the traffic. Henry and Jack were home in Washington with my mother and father. For the time being, everything was out of my control.

I called Northwest Airlines three different times to be sure Allen's flight had taken off and landed safely. As on so many previous days, sporting my running shoes, I started walking and followed the green lights through the streets of New York. I wandered aimlessly and quietly, as this was pre-iPod times, stopping for a piece of Godiva chocolate on Madison Avenue, always resisting the urge to wander into Baby Gap, though I did look in the windows. As the day passed, I got more and more anxious about the decisions we might have to make. Dr. Hughes had less than forty-eight hours to test the cells. If he had confidence in the HLA and FA test results, the decision would be easy: implant the one, two, or three healthy HLA matches; and freeze the others for future use. We flat-out dismissed our families' and friends' concerns about what in the world we would do with triplets. We were too focused on what we would do without Henry.

It was possible, however, that Dr. Hughes could be sure about the FA diagnosis or the HLA diagnosis, but not about both. It was possible that we could be faced with a decision to implant embryos that were definitely HLA matches, but where the disease status was unclear. I wasn't sure I could bear yet another trimester of pregnancy not knowing whether our baby had FA. It was possible that if we took that chance and implanted two embryos, I could get pregnant with twins, both of whom would be HLA matches, but one of whom could have FA. Then we would have to consider having selective reduction, a process where the growth of the diseased fetus could be terminated while preserving the remaining healthy one. What if we did that and they terminated the wrong one? Walking the streets of New York, I thought about how I had once imagined my life as a parent; how simple I thought it would be back on that October day six years earlier, when Allen slipped the *Laurie Will You Marry Me? Please Say Yes!* mix tape into the tape deck.

Up until Henry's birth, my life had been so easy. For the most part, I made the team, secured the invitation, got the guy. My life was like a piñata—good things just kept coming out. Most days I had woken up with a feeling of excitement, as if something good was going to happen and I had to get up and get out of the house to find out what it was. One of those days, Allen and I decided to wake up together every day and see what great things we could make happen if we combined our optimism, energy, and appetite for fun.

That our first big production, our first baby, came with so much hardship, so early in our relationship, was still incomprehensible to me.

Henry's prognosis, his open-heart surgery, these high-stakes attempts at PGD brought out unfamiliar emotions—fear, helplessness, vulnerability, depression. We were unpracticed at discussing such complex emotional matters with each other, or with our friends and family. Our hardship quickly revealed new and uncomfortable needs: money to help pay for medical treatments and to support research; people willing to sign up as potential bone-marrow donors; family and friends to provide practical, day-to-day help and extraordinary and enduring amounts of comfort and compassion.

How the hell had my life gotten so complicated? I longed for the day when I could take the kids to the park, have a picnic, and worry about what they ate for lunch or where I should send them to summer camp. I longed for the day when I could stop worrying about platelet counts, CBCs, and HLA matches.

Late that night, Allen returned from his trip to Detroit. Having seen Dr. Hughes for the first time in a year and a half doubly reinforced his confidence. Henry may have been Batman, but when Dr. Hughes donned his lab coat, to Allen he was none other than Superman. Two days later, we went to Cornell hospital three times for our embryo transfer. Twice we were sent away and told to return later, as Dr. Hughes had not yet called Drs. Rosenwaks and Xu in New York with the test results. Sometime after six p.m., we returned to the hospital and I changed into a hospital gown, slippers, and a hairnet so I would be ready as soon as they got the call from Dr. Hughes. The embryos had been growing in a lab outside my body for several days, and it was time to put them back in to ensure that they would develop into a baby.

After I dressed, Allen and I took a seat in the surgical waiting room, which, with its pink walls and circular shape, felt to me like a throwback to the 1950s. A few other couples had come and gone, and it was starting to get late. Finally, Dr. Xu, the embryologist, entered.

"Mark Hughes wants to talk to you," he said. Allen got on the phone right away. I could tell by looking at his face that something was wrong. Allen hung up and took my hands.

"Just tell me," I said.

"Of the sixteen embryos, two are perfect HLA matches."

"That's great!" I said, feeling a surge of enormous relief that in a flash was tempered by the sad look in Allen's eyes. "That's great, right?"

"Laurie. I'm so sorry. They both have Fanconi."

I collapsed on the floor, naked except for the gown. I couldn't bear to look at Allen. I couldn't bear to get up. So I just lay there, curled around myself, wishing I could get smaller and smaller until there was nothing left.

*F*or the next six months, we waited. Claudia Hughes was fighting for her life and Dr. Hughes was at her bedside. He also wanted to spend time understanding what had happened with our case to see what he could learn to improve the outcome the next time. In the meantime, we continued to organize bone-marrow drives and to try to convince the insurance company to pay for our PGD attempts. Initially they refused to cover PGD on the basis that they didn't cover treatment for infertility. When we pointed out that our two children were proof that we weren't infertile and that they should cover PGD as a bone-marrow donor search, they reiterated their refusal to cover treatment for infertility and added that they cover only donor searches outside of the family. Despite the letters we submitted from our doctors who, among other things, explained that the cost of a transplant with the marrow of a stranger far exceeded (perhaps by more than 100 percent) the cost of one with the perfect sibling donor produced through PGD, the insurance company steadfastly refused. It was as if they had never heard of PGD. I found that if I submitted my bills for everything except the $250 quarterly fee for frozen embryo storage, sometimes they would cover blood tests and sonograms; other times, the cost of the anesthesia. It didn't amount to much, but we would take what we could get, and our extended family made up the difference, for which we are eternally grateful.

Despite the devastating results, the progress we had made in our second PGD attempt combined with the fact that we had no other options solidified our belief that it was well worth waiting for a third try when Dr. Hughes was ready for us. In the meantime, we were hardly going to sit around and let life pass us by. In July 1998, the four of us, along with my parents and Allen's parents, traveled to a small fishing village in Galicia, Spain, to attend the wedding of Allen's best friend, Bill Delaney, to his fiancée, Cristina Alvarez.

From the moment we stepped onboard the flight to Spain, we got the vacation we had been hoping for and so desperately needed. Henry spent the six-hour flight running up and down the aisles, making friends and on occasion getting someone to play Go Fish with him. Compliments of the pilot, who was a friend of Cristina's, my dad—who, in addition to being a lawyer and sailor, is also a pilot—was invited to sit in the cockpit for the takeoff from Dulles Airport. The trip would prove to be filled with similar treats for all of us.

Laguardia, the town where we stayed, was postcard-perfect. It is tiny and hilly, with narrow streets that draw very few tourists. Nobody spoke a word of English. Along the harbor were rows of small restaurants with langostinos and fresh catch hanging in the window like the ducks beckoning diners in Chinatown.

It was sunny and warm, and in the afternoons, we'd all go swimming in the cool, blue waters of the Atlantic Ocean, waiting for the fishermen to pull their boats into the little harbor. They'd carry the day's catch into an airy brick building and pour their piles of still-squirming fish—squid, octopus, and so many things we couldn't identify—onto the floor. Local restaurateurs and housewives would arrive, carrying their baskets and bags, and cart away their pick. Henry loved it. He'd stoop down low to inspect the strange creatures while Jack, after taking one look at a big octopus, let out a shriek and ran for the door. He would carry a fear of octopus with him for a long time: a pretty significant inconvenience for Jack, a lover of wildlife and marine animals.

We got lucky one afternoon and came upon a festival at the dock. "See if you can find us," Henry called from a beautiful wooden boat where he and Jack hid. A balloon artist made Henry and me silly blue, red, and purple balloon hats that we wore as we held hands and sat on a wall above the ocean. The boys played soccer in the courtyard of the Convento de San Benito, a convent that had been converted to a hotel, where Allen's and my parents were staying.

One day we joined my parents and the bride and groom on a boat trip to remote islands off the coast of Portugal for swimming and a seafood feast. "No boat, no boat!" Jack cried, an hour into a daylong trip. Henry, a year older and a lot more adventurous, asked the captain if he could wear his hat and steer the boat. The next day, after a lengthy bus trip to the magnificent Santiago de Compostela cathedral in Northwest Spain, Jack cried, "No bus, no bus!" "No (insert transportation mode)" remains part of our family lexicon.

One evening, the grandparents looked after Henry and Jack while Allen and I joined Bill and Cristina on a drive through the vineyard-dotted countryside. It was a beautiful night as we pulled up in front of what looked like two huge boulders in the middle of nowhere. There were no people. No signs. No thoughts of IVF or PGD. Just an opening in the rocks, and then a serene, romantic restaurant called La Gare. It was in a private home, with a three-hundred-year-old wine press on-site, and the whole place was lit only by candles.

The owner, who greeted and served us, grew up in the house. He brought to our table dishes of the freshest, most delicious food I'd ever tasted: roasted peppers, fish, local *tetilla* cheese. Grapes hung from the lattice above, we drank wine, and as I watched Allen in the shadow of the candlelight, enjoying our friends, looking forward to the wedding, I felt so happy; at peace, even. Those were feelings I wasn't sure I'd ever feel again. But it stayed with me for those days we had together in Spain—ten days during which I enjoyed my friends, spoiled my kids, and relished the freedom of not having to fight for a thing.

Henry's Favorite Things

- Making snowmen
- Riding the black panther on the Central
  Park carousel
- Going to Disney World
- Visits from the Happy Heartbeat clowns,
  including Dr. Jill E. Bean and
  Dr. Chick 'N Pox
- When Snow White says, "You must be Grumpy"
- Riding in Nana's Mustang convertible
- Reading *Encyclopedia Brown* and solving the crime

8

DWELLING IN POSSIBILITY

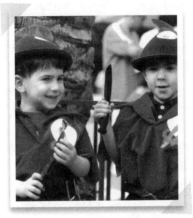

*Henry and Jack ready for battle with
Captain Hook*

"*J*ake loves sports," said his mom, Helaine. "Especially baseball and the Baltimore Orioles."

It was the fall of 1998, a few months after returning from Spain, and Allen and I were at parents' night at the beginning of Henry's first year in preschool. A group of about twenty-five moms and dads sat on small blue plastic chairs arranged in a circle. I sat next to the cubbies, each carefully labeled with a student's name and his or her photo, and filled with a change of clothes and some extra diapers and wipes. Henry's cubby featured a photo of him riding the black panther on the carousel in Central Park. Like many preschool classrooms, the bulletin boards were covered with the letters of the alphabet and colorful photographs. The bookshelves were filled with classics, like *The Three Billy Goats Gruff* and *Where the Wild Things Are.* There was a dress-up corner with costumes, and an art table overflowing with paints and brushes, markers, and Play-Doh.

Henry's teacher Liane, Bella's mom, had welcomed us, and suggested that we each share something special about our child to help us get to know one another.

Susan went next. "Simon loves cars."

"So does Ari," Linda said.

Perhaps they'll be friends, I thought.

I looked around. Everyone was smiling and dressed beautifully. Some mothers were pregnant, and others had clearly lost their pregnancy weight. I had just learned that I was not pregnant following my third PGD attempt, though thanks to the bloating from the months of injections, I looked as if I might be.

It would soon be our turn to speak. My heart started beating fast and my palms started to sweat. I wanted to grab Allen and run. This was yet another place where we did not belong.

"Eyal is great at puzzles. He is up to two hundred pieces," said his mother. "He and Jake have been best friends since they were born, and they are so excited to be in class together," she added.

One after another, mothers and fathers shared something wonderful or ordinary about their sons and daughters. As I listened, I wondered which of these children Henry would befriend, and if there was another mom sitting around the circle who could possibly relate to what I was going through.

Then it was my turn. I paused and looked around the room.

What could I say? The first thing that came to my mind was: *Everything. Everything about Henry is special.*

But I couldn't say that. I couldn't say any of the things that came to me:

Henry is brave. He brings a sword with him to the doctor each week when he gets his blood checked. He looks at the nurse, smiles, and says, "Bring it on."

Henry has a rare, fatal disease.

Henry might die before he gets to kindergarten.

"Henry loves Batman." This is what I said out loud.

Henry also loved school. Each morning, he would jump out of bed, excited for whatever the day would bring. He especially loved Circle Time, where he could share lucky pennies, new Batman and Pokémon figures, or feathers and other cool stuff he had found at his grandparents' home on Maryland's Eastern Shore.

On the first day of the school year, Liane and her co-teacher, Denis, sent the first of many notes home. "Henry had a GREAT first day!" they said. He had drawn a picture of himself with his three new friends: Jake, Simon, and Ari, who would become his friends for life, just as their parents would become ours. Henry played baseball with Jake, cars with Ari, and Pokémon with Simon. Often after school, they would go together with their nannies to nearby Macomb Park to climb on the spiderweb or play soccer; to Turtle Park to play in the sandbox, treehouse or the sprinkler; or to one another's houses for lunch.

And within days, Henry had met and fallen in love with Bella.

Henry's preschool classroom was hardly the only venue where I felt out of place. As Allen and I struggled with what we were going through, and with the knowledge that while Henry seemed fine, his healthy days were numbered, I began to feel so completely alone.

I tried my best to make it different. I'd do everything I could to make sure I didn't miss a dinner with the Ladies of the Pines, despite how lousy or disappointed I felt when the evening to meet rolled around. And while I was there at the table with my friends and I laughed along with their stories, I just couldn't relate. Not to the tales of new boyfriends, bad or lost jobs, money. By this time, our group had expanded beyond the original BOA; while two other women were married, most were not, and only one had a child. Certainly no one else had a child with a fatal disease.

Nobody ever intended me to feel left out—and it would probably have killed them to know how I felt—but my circumstances did leave me out. All I could think was that I wasn't fun anymore, that I was a huge bummer, and they probably didn't even want me around because all I did was bring everyone down. It was such a weird role for me. Prior to Henry's diagnosis, I had been the crazy one of the group: among the most outgoing, the most up for adventure, the one trying to talk everyone else into removing their clothes and running along the Beltway with me. And now here I was, barely able to add anything to the conversation happening around the table. All I seemed to know how to talk about anymore was my state of desperation.

But sometimes, despite even the best intentions, people did do or say things that hurt me so much, or, worse, made me feel misunderstood or transparent. During a dinner with some newer friends, the conversation turned to a story about some mutual friends who had just given birth to a child who was ill. I didn't say anything, I just listened as they talked about how our friends would never be happy again. They vocalized their concerns about what if something like that ever happened to them. *It would be terrible. It would ruin my life.* I sat there debating whether I should just get up and leave,

tell them how what they were saying made me feel, or try to lend
whatever insight and experience I had. I opted for the third option
and said that although it was true that our friends' lives and dreams
for their child would have to be altered, I bet that they could find
happiness. I bet they would learn to change their expectations. They
would learn how to get a whole lot of good out of almost each and
every day. This was a big step for me, but I didn't feel as if they heard
what I was saying and the conversation steered back to "what if" it
happened to them.

I stopped going to those dinners after that.

*H*enry, on the other hand, never talked about his sickness. In
fact, he didn't seem to know he was sick, nor did any of his friends.
Their parents found out over time. Once, when we were playing in
the sprinkler at nearby Turtle Park, Henry took off his shirt, reveal-
ing the long, jagged scar down his chest, compliments of his open-
heart surgery. That's how Simon's mom, Susan, found out.

Before or after school once a week, and sometimes more often
than that, Henry would visit his doctor and give a couple of vials of
blood so the doctor could check to see if he had enough white blood
cells to fight germs, or if his platelet count was high enough to ensure that his blood would clot properly if he fell and got cut. Sometimes he would miss a few days of school because he had to travel to
New Jersey to visit Dr. Gillio and undergo anesthesia and a bone-
marrow aspiration and biopsy to see how his disease was progressing, and how much more time we had prior to his inevitable
bone-marrow transplant. Henry wore more Band-Aids than most
kids, and from time to time, it occurred to me that the growing
number of black-and-blue marks that covered his arms, legs, and
face as a result of a low platelet count might raise questions. But he
could run and play as well, if not better, than other kids his age.

I knew that being a good mom to Henry meant letting Henry just be Henry. This meant, for example, that I took a front-row seat as Henry began to engage Jack in an intense training regimen. They started out with wrestling. They wrestled in their bedrooms, in forts they made in the basement, on Allen's and my bed, and in the backyard. They were like two tiger cubs rolled into a ball, covered with dirt or grass or leaves. As they got older, they turned to swordfighting. In our living room, they each donned a silver helmet, chest piece, shield, plastic blunt-tipped sword, and sheath. Jack started hitting Henry's sword. "Jack, take the cover off first," Henry explained. Jack did as he was told, and they got to work. "Huh! Huh! Huh! Huh! Huh!" they each shouted as their swords slapped against each other. "Gotcha!" said Henry as he stuck his sword under Jack's chest piece.

While Henry noticed the bruises these activities left on him, he never asked why he had to go to the doctor more often than Jack or anyone else. It was just part of his routine, along with going to school, soccer practice, or swimming lessons. If you saw us eating ice-cream cones at Max's Ice Cream, or riding the carousel at Glen Echo Park, or playing in the surf at the beach, you would think we were just another happy family.

Knowing from our third attempt that we could produce healthy HLA matches through PGD motivated us to return to New York as soon as possible to try again. So in November 1998, I traveled to New York for my fourth attempt. A few days after I arrived, Henry, who had just turned three, had an appointment in Hackensack for his semiannual bone-marrow aspiration. This procedure allowed Dr. Gillio to look for any evidence of life-threatening disease like leukemia, which in Henry's case was a sure death sentence. No one with Fanconi anemia whose bone-marrow failure had led to leukemia prior to having a bone-marrow transplant had ever survived the transplant, regardless of the donor. I raced out of the IVF clinic in New York City, armed with doughnuts, chocolate milk, and coffee, and arrived in Hackensack just in time. I always held Henry as the anesthetic was inserted into his IV, so he could fall asleep in my arms.

That day we learned that Henry's platelets had fallen dramatically to 19,000—their lowest ever. When they dropped to 10,000, Henry would need a transfusion. The news threatened to push me over the edge. The drugs I had been taking for nearly a year at this point had ravaged me—physically and emotionally—and I didn't know if I was strong enough to handle yet another setback in a long string of failures. I never had time to recover from one before the next one struck. While Allen stayed with Henry and Jack, I walked out of the clinic doors and through the winding hallways I knew so well to the lobby. I got a cup of coffee and settled into one of the big chairs facing outside and took a deep breath, fighting the tears. I hated this. I hated Fanconi anemia and hospitals and needles and drugs. I hated all the waiting for appointments, tests, results, good news and bad news, over and over again. I hated all of it.

But with the news we'd just heard (*19,000*—I couldn't get it out of my head), I didn't have the option of taking a break or having a breakdown. I didn't even allow myself to cry. If Henry was just months away from requiring a transplant, then this was nothing compared to what awaited us. Besides, I needed to be the strong one. At this stage, the success of the PGD—and Henry's life—depended on me. I walked back to the clinic, regaining a little more of my composure and resolve with each step. An hour later, we were at Short Hills Mall drinking chocolate milkshakes, listening to Elvis Presley's "Hound Dog" on the jukebox at Johnny Rockets, and heavily engaged in Batman versus Power Rangers battles.

That afternoon, while Allen and the boys took naps, I lay on the couch trying to find peace, and the energy and optimism I would need to make it through my egg retrieval that week. The nurse at Cornell eventually called to let me know that I needed to return to the clinic that very evening for another sonogram to help Dr. Rosenwaks decide whether I should take hCG that night. So by seven thirty p.m., I was back in the car, driving to New York City for the second time that day. Thinking ahead, I brought my pajamas, some Lupron, some Follistim, some hCG, and a bunch of needles, prepared for whatever the night would bring. Allen stayed behind with the boys. It was important to us that they had at least one parent with them whenever possible.

I met one of the IVF nurses and went up to the clinic to join Dr. Rosenwaks. It was empty, other than the cleaning crew. Dr. Rosenwaks determined that I would have to take the hCG at one thirty a.m. and then return to the clinic for preop, bloodwork, and a sonogram between seven and eight thirty a.m. Too tired to drive anywhere, let alone coordinate logistics, I decided to stay in my aunt and uncle's new apartment in New York City, which was too small to accommodate my family but was perfect for me. I just needed to figure out who could give me the hCG, an injection that required putting a very long needle into my hard-to-reach-myself rear end. Half-joking, I wondered aloud to the nurse if giving shots to residents' relatives was part of the doorman's job description. The nurse gave me quick instructions in the self-administration of subcutaneous shots and drew a target with black magic marker on my skin so I would know exactly where to aim the two-inch needle. I walked through the empty fertility clinic, took the elevator downstairs, and walked back to the apartment in the darkness of the night.

When the alarm went off at 1:20 a.m., I was alone and confused. Within minutes, the phone rang. Allen was on the other end, calling to make sure I was awake and to talk me through the shot. I walked sleepily to the bathroom and turned on the light, my feet cold on the tiled floor. Blearily, I read the instructions for the hCG several times out loud, so tired that I feared that I was incapable of following directions, wondering if I was truly awake or just dreaming.

"You can do this," Allen said encouragingly. "You've had to do a lot worse."

After a cold splash of water, I focused, picked up the first syringe, and prepared the injection. My stomach hurt. It was one thing to inject the needle in my thighs, as I had more than a hundred times before, but this needle was thicker and longer, and its destination was nearly inaccessible. I had never before had to administer it myself.

Time was running out. "I'm gonna do it," I said to Allen. I put the phone down.

As the clock turned to 1:30 a.m., I reached around and aimed for the target. I pushed the needle through my skin. Switching to my left hand, I used my right hand to slowly pull back on the syringe to make sure I hadn't hit a blood vessel. There was no blood in the syringe, so I pushed it all the way in and then quickly pulled it out. Relieved, exhausted, and impressed, I said good night to Allen and went back to the bed to lie down, only to be awakened five hours later by an alarm clock, sounding the need to return to the clinic for my preop visit. I gave blood, got a sonogram, got my egg-retrieval instructions, and headed to New Jersey to return the car to Allen and say good-bye to him and the kids, who would drive home later that day.

After we parted, I fell into a deep sleep, woke up, and went to the train station headed for Manhattan so I could get to the apartment and try to sleep some more. After driving the four hours home, Allen was joined by my mom, who would spend the night, allowing Allen to turn right back around at six the next morning to catch the train back to New York and be with me for the egg retrieval. Besides wanting to keep each other company through such hard times, Allen had to provide fresh semen to fertilize the eggs.

I awoke from the anesthesia to hear the nurse muttering an awesome pair of words: "Thirty eggs."

Three days later, Allen flew to Detroit with biopsied cells from twenty-one of them. Two days later in Manhattan, we learned by cell phone on the corner of Eighty-second Street and Third Avenue that out of the twenty-one embryos, we did not get one single healthy match.

"I'm so, so sorry," Allen said after hanging up. "But we have time to do it again. Let's call Dr. Rosenwaks's office and make an appointment. This can still work. I know it's hard, especially on you, but we have no other option."

"That's easy for you to say!" I yelled. "My body is ravaged. I'm covered with bruises, bloated, miserable, and I feel like shit. All you have to do is look at *Playboy* and masturbate." Without saying another word, we went to Penn Station and boarded a train for home. I almost wished it would just run off the tracks and put an end to the whole damn thing. Around the time the train approached the station in Metropark, New Jersey, Allen reached into his backpack and pulled out a book of photos he kept with him when he traveled. Henry and Jack on a carousel, in a pumpkin patch, on the soccer field, laughing their heads off with brownie mix all over their faces. By the time we got home, I couldn't wait to get back to New York to try yet again.

*D*r. Hughes's wife died after an agonizing battle with cancer during the week of the egg retrieval in my fifth PGD attempt. Allen flew with Dr. Rosenwaks to Detroit for her funeral. Since my ovaries were well into egg production, we were beyond the point of no return, so we had to proceed with the retrieval, without knowing if the genetic testing would occur. We discussed two options with Dr. Rosenwaks. They could retrieve the eggs and fertilize them, after which they would immediately be frozen prior to any cell division. Theoretically, they could be thawed and biopsied when Dr. Hughes's lab was ready to do the diagnostic work. This option significantly extended the uncertainty. The second option was to go ahead with the entire procedure with Dr. Hughes's lab staff, but without Dr. Hughes. He had a committed and talented staff, but he was the expert, and ours was such a significant case, and one in which he was so personally invested. After all this time, and all that we had been through together, it didn't seem right to move forward without our partner.

On February 10, 1999, the doctor retrieved seventeen eggs. I balanced being disappointed at the comparatively low number I had produced with my understanding that the numbers hadn't really mattered much in the past. Of those, seven were robust and were suitable for testing. I was convinced this would be a bust just like all the others. Although I tried to find some hope within, the road had been too long and too hard, with too many disappointments. I was sick and tired of false hope.

Two days later, Dr. Hughes, who had found a way to help us in the midst of his own terrible loss, called to say we had one healthy, HLA match that was not very good quality. There was also another one that was a great embryo, healthy with a 50 percent chance of being a perfect HLA match. After all these attempts (we now had created seventy embryos), we had only produced four healthy, HLA matches—none of which were good-quality embryos. I reasoned that for this to work, we would probably have to take a risk and implant an embryo that we weren't 100 percent sure was a perfect HLA match, but that actually had a chance at producing a pregnancy. We weren't willing to take a risk and implant an embryo that might have Fanconi, but implanting one that might not be an HLA match was different because the baby would be healthy. Because the embryo quality was good, I could get pregnant with a healthy baby that could turn out to be a genetic mismatch. An embryo that had 50 percent chance of being an HLA match was a lot more promising than one with the 18.75 percent chance that we could produce on our own. But, if I got pregnant with a mismatch and carried the pregnancy to term, we would run out of time to help Henry. Could we really decide to roll the dice after all that we had been through?

We had fifteen minutes to decide.

*W*e couldn't do it. We just couldn't risk the chance that despite everything that we had gone through, Henry could still die. Although I was wavering, Allen was adamant. Go with the one that we are certain about and if it doesn't produce a pregnancy, we can come back and do it all over again. Again, easy for him to say. We taped the picture of embryo 11—a craggly, circular shape with textures and bubbles, like the surface of the moon—on the dashboard of our car and drove back to Washington.

Two weeks later, I got up early the morning of my pregnancy test scheduled at a fertility clinic near our home in D.C. Henry was already awake, so I brought him along for good luck.

Later that afternoon, we were at my parents' house. Allen was so confident that I was pregnant that he thought we should call the doctor's office for the results with everyone around us. In my parents' kitchen, Allen dialed the doctor's office on speakerphone.

A nurse told us that I wasn't pregnant. She was genuinely sorry. I was genuinely angry. Not at her or anyone in particular, but at the whole thing.

"I'm sick of feeling sick and tired," I told Allen angrily as my parents quickly ushered the kids out of the room and out of earshot. "I'm sick of being separated from you and the boys. I'm sick of having my hopes raised and then dashed. I'm sick of the whole damn thing."

Allen didn't dare try to convince me that things were going to be OK this time. I looked him in the eye. "Face it," I said, "this is never, ever, ever going to work. I will do it again and again because we have no other options. But we both know it is never going to work."

"Let's go home," Allen said despondently.

On the way home, Allen put a Disney CD on the car stereo and Jack and Henry, ages two and three, strapped into their car seats in the back, started singing the lyrics to "You've Got a Friend in Me," from the movie *Toy Story*. They were both smiling, flashing their dimples, kicking their legs, looking like they didn't have a care in the world. I glanced into the backseat at them and allowed myself to revel in their purity and innocence. I turned to Allen and said quietly, "I'm so sorry. I can do this. It has to work. I'm not going to let him die."

*M*ore than 175 shots, 97 eggs, and 4 potential, but failed, pregnancies later, we were no closer to saving Henry's life than we were eighteen months earlier when we took our first step down this path. We could now officially say that we had done everything we could to help Henry. But that was little solace.

Later that night, I sent an e-mail to the Nashes to let them know that things hadn't worked out for us yet again. I know how difficult that news had to be for them to receive, as Molly's platelet count was falling and they had waited a long time for us to achieve success that only seemed to evade us. Dr. Hughes was still waiting to be successful with us prior to offering this service to other couples. That week, Allen had seen an article on the Internet that mentioned a doctor in Baltimore who might be doing work similar to Dr. Hughes's, and he passed that information along to the Nashes. They had also contacted a doctor in Chicago whom they thought could help them.

Meanwhile, we dug deep within ourselves to explore our alternatives. We could give up on the preimplantation genetic diagnosis. Clearly things were not working out the way we hoped or planned. We reexplored the survival rate for nonsibling, matched bone-marrow donors, hoping that in the more than three years since we began to pursue this treatment, perhaps things had improved. We learned that the survival rate for unrelated (nonsibling) donor transplants for the type of Fanconi anemia that Henry had was still zero. You'd have to be pretty darn lucky to defy those odds. While there was once a time when I considered myself a lucky person, that felt like a very long time ago.

There were two remaining options: Give up on PGD and get pregnant on our own, with the hope that we get the break that had eluded us for years, or continue doing PGD. The more Allen and I talked about what we had been through, the more we knew that we couldn't abandon our efforts. But next time, we would broaden what was acceptable for embryo transfer to include those that were Fanconi-free and had at least a 50 percent chance of being a genetic match, as opposed to being a perfect match. If Dr. Hughes was sure that one or more embryos matched the HLA type that *either* Allen or I passed on to Henry, and that the other half of the HLA match was uncertain, we would take our chances and implant. Although that meant that we wouldn't know if we were successful until I was near the end of my first trimester, we would have a much better chance than we would on our own. This way we would be assured that the baby was healthy, the most critical factor, and that we had a good chance of saving Henry's life.

After the series of long, difficult conversations it took to finally arrive at this course of action, Allen and I made one more very important decision.

.   .   .

"We're going where?" Jack yelled.

"You heard her," Henry said. "We're going to Disney World!"

It was a few weeks later, and two volunteers from the Make-A-Wish Foundation were in our dining room, along with my parents, Allen's parents, Abby and her family, Andrew and his family, a bunch of balloons, a very large cake, and two little boys, wearing their brand-new Mickey Mouse ears and smiles big enough to light up all of Washington.

We hadn't told Henry or Jack of the timing of this trip, but it originated during an interview Henry had with two Make-A-Wish volunteers that Allen had organized. The volunteers had posed the question, "If you could go anywhere or do anything you wanted, what would you choose?" Clearly they got the message.

Within days, the four of us were bound for Orlando, Florida. We spent a week at the park, beginning each day with the all-you-can-eat breakfast with the Disney characters and ending it crowded together, watching the late-night fireworks. Henry's special distinction as a Make-A-Wish guest meant that we never waited in any lines for rides (they thoughtfully usher you in through the exit) or to meet the Disney characters. Henry and Jack rode roller coasters; bought new costumes and dressed up as Buzz Lightyear, Peter Pan, and Captain Hook; met and dined with Mickey and Minnie Mouse, Peter Pan, Snow White, Cinderella, and dozens of other characters; and filled autograph books and photo albums.

Whenever Henry saw one of the Disney characters, he would grab his autograph book and run as fast as he could to meet them. In contrast, Jack would run in the opposite direction. "Mom, Tigger is after me. Help me!" he yelled as he catapulted into my arms. After Henry secured each autograph, he would give the character a huge hug, wrapping his small arms as far as he could around their waists. Pictures from the trip feature Henry hugging Mickey Mouse, Henry hugging Cinderella, Henry hugging Mary Poppins, Peter Pan, Chip,

Dale, Snow White, and Buzz Lightyear. We spent several days chasing after Snow White, who threatened to steal Henry's heart from his lifelong love, his girlfriend, Bella.

"Mom, can I see Snow White again?" he asked within an hour of seeing her. We eventually found her by Cinderella's Castle. "Mom, can I see Snow White again?" repeated Henry after she left. After searching nearly every square foot of the Magic Kingdom, Henry settled on a Snow White doll.

Enamored with dressing up, Henry and Jack each acquired a Peter Pan costume and a green felt hat with their name sewn on it adorned with a red feather. One evening at a Disney character dinner at the Grand Floridian Hotel, our two little Peter Pans were surprised and delighted to meet the *real* Peter Pan. After autographs and hugs and the third ice cream of the day, we left, and Henry and Jack came upon a little boy dressed as Captain Hook in the garden outside the hotel. The three of them held an impromptu sword fight. Knocking the laughing Hook's sword out of his hand, Jack exclaimed, "I got him, Henry! I got him!"

"Good job, honey," I called to Jack, as all three kids romped around the garden.

If only all of Henry's enemies could be so easily vanquished.

Henry's Favorite Things

- Disney character breakfasts and dinners
- Blasting stomp rockets over our neighbor's house
- Anything "rare"
- Playing hide-and-seek
- Parades
- Magic tricks
- Magic Markers

9

It's a Wrap

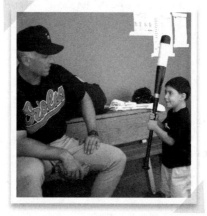

Henry gives Cal Ripken Jr. batting tips

*U*nfortunately, our escape from reality would only be temporary. A month after we returned home from Florida, in June 1999, I found myself once again in New York, standing alone before two vials and two syringes, preparing to inject hCG into the black target drawn on my skin. In addition to the fact that Allen and I had already decided that this time—our sixth PGD attempt—we were willing to transfer HLA-uncertain, but potentially lifesaving, healthy embryos, Dr. Hughes had also told us of a promising new development: He had worked out an alternative method of interpreting the HLA type, which would increase the certainty of the genetic diagnosis.

The next day I awoke from a drug-induced sedation to hear the nurse telling me that they had retrieved twenty-eight eggs. Finally, I thought, our tenacity had paid off.

Allen and I were eating our typical breakfast—scrambled eggs and rye toast—in our booth at EJ's Luncheonette on Seventy-third and Third the next day when an IVF nurse called with our fertilization results. Of the twenty-eight eggs, only fourteen fertilized. Overnight, our chance of success was cut in half. Over the din of plates being cleared and silverware clanging, I asked the nurse if she was sure she was reading Laurie Strongin's chart.

"I want to go home," I said to Allen, as soon as I hung up.

"Are you sure?"

"Yes. The thought of hanging around for another four days of building anxiety, leading up to a crescendo of bad news . . . it's too much for me to bear. I need to see Henry and Jack. Let's all get our lives back, if only for a few days."

And so we went. The next morning I woke up in my own bed, made the boys breakfast, and squandered an afternoon at the park—an act of normalcy that I cherished. I spent the day as I usually did: mastering the art of timing Henry's and Jack's swings just right so I could push one while the other was swinging at his peak. By this time, Jack had gone from being Henry's plaything to his favorite playmate. Decked out in capes and masks, Henry and Jack were the Caped Crusaders of our Glover Park neighborhood. Henry, of course, was Batman. These days, I reveled in the simple act of watching my boys being children. Jack would walk into the kitchen in a well-worn hand-me-down Batman costume, only to appear, an hour later, in his new bright red-and-green Robin costume. I'd listen to them playing hide-and-seek in the living room in the evenings as we waited for Allen to come home and I set our table for dinner. Jack's strategy was genius: He'd sit on the couch and put his hands over his eyes. Clearly, if he couldn't see anyone, they couldn't see him. Henry played along. He'd walk into the kitchen, flash me a big grin.

"I wonder where Jack is?" he'd say. "Could he be under the kitchen table? Nope." He'd disappear and I'd hear him calling out from the other rooms of the house. "Could he be in the closet? No. Could he be in the bathtub? No. Where could he be?"

Finally, Jack would remove his fingers from his face, and call out, exasperated: "Here I am, Henry! Over here!"

Heroes and their sidekicks often have differing strengths, and that was certainly true for Henry and Jack. Athletic by nature, Henry was a star on the Dolphins team in his soccer league, and a champion monkey-bar navigator. Jack, far more cerebral and limitlessly curious, was our Boy Wonder. He spent much of his time on the soccer field looking for four-leaf clovers and identifying shapes made out of clouds. Shortly after mastering Dr. Seuss, Jack would move on to encyclopedias, learning and amassing an incredible and varied set of facts about subjects ranging from animals to superheroes, geography to world history, mythology to religion. "Ask Jack," was the answer to nearly any question that anyone asked the three of us. Clearly if any of us needed a lifeline, we had someone to call.

Two days after we returned from New York, Allen was on the 7:00 a.m. train, heading back. Once there, he retrieved the cells from the ten remaining embryos at Weill Cornell, jumped in a cab, and boarded a flight bound for Detroit. He had dinner with Dr. Hughes and his children, who were teenagers at the time, before returning to BWI to arrive home around one thirty a.m. The next morning, Allen and I drove together to New York City for our test results. Two hundred and thirty miles is a long way to go for a phone call—especially one that in the past had so often brought bad news. But we had to be near the hospital so that, in the event of good news, we could do the embryo transfer immediately. As had become the custom, my mother stayed with Henry and Jack for the two days we would be in Manhattan completing the PGD cycle. As our sons understood it, our trips to New York were to go to the doctor so that we could someday bring back a baby brother or sister. In the meantime, we would return armed with Batman figurines for each of them.

After lunch, our cell phone rang. I fished it out of my purse and handed it to Allen. I saw the glimmer of a smile followed by Allen's first-class dimples, then quickly handed him a pen and paper. I eagerly read what he was scribbling: "recommendation no disease; half HLA match; 65% sure identical; 1 great; 1 pretty good; if they take have greater than 50% chance."

The translation: FINALLY!!

Of the ten embryos tested, two were healthy and had the HLA typing that Allen gave Henry. Dr. Hughes was 65 percent sure that they got the HLA typing that I gave Henry, but this part wasn't definitive. Of the two, one was a great-quality embryo, something we had never had before; the other was pretty good.

With tears running down my face and Allen's hand gripped tightly in mine, we ran for the car and drove to the hospital at Sixty-eighth and York. This was it. Assembled in the operating room were Dr. Rosenwaks and a colleague, along with Dr. Xu and Ruby, the nurse who had been by my side during each and every procedure, ushering in our dream.

Ten days later, I was sort of pregnant. My test was positive, but my hormone level was very low. I would have to repeat the test two days later. Unfortunately, I was scheduled to leave for Chicago the next day for a work event that I had been planning for months on predatory lending and its ill effects on low-income families and communities.

At seven a.m. on the day of my event, I took a cab to a local Chicago hospital to have my blood drawn by someone who didn't know how much I needed good news. Oddly enough, Lisa Nash was presently undergoing PGD at the same hospital, having found other doctors to help her. In the cab back to the hotel, I leaned my head against the window, watched the city pass by, and hoped beyond hope for good news. I was bone-tired, partly because of the travel, and partly because of all the energy I devoted to hoping for success. Since starting PGD, we'd never had this good a chance, and deep inside I believed that this time, it was going to work. The doctors I had been speaking to over the last few days had all gently warned me not to get my hopes up too high. Based on the results of the test I had taken two days earlier, they said it didn't look promising. But as I slipped out of the cab that morning and headed to the meeting, I pushed aside their words of caution and the fact that, even in the best of circumstances, IVF works only one-third of the time.

Maybe I was crazy, maybe I was stubborn. But either way, I held on to the hope. It was the only thing I had left.

I wasn't pregnant.

I was told this news on a pay phone, in the hallway of the hotel, where, in the conference room next door, hundreds of strangers were gathered. I barely remember that day, which melted into a blur of sadness, anger, and devastating disappointment; and a need for me to do my job, to act like a normal person with a normal life, able to carry on normal conversations and care about things that were not matters of life or death. It was almost more than I could handle.

· · ·

$\mathcal{B}$ut there was more. *The seventh attempt.* The night when Allen had to drive six hundred miles on four hours' sleep from New York to Detroit through the eye of Hurricane Floyd, the cells in a cooler in the backseat of a rental car, after his flight was cancelled.

The eighth attempt; the morning I found out I was pregnant. With an HLA-match. Finally pregnant.

"It's all been worth it," I had told my parents over the phone, all of us too overcome with joy and emotion to say much more. Then I handed the phone to Allen, who sat next to me at the desk in his office, as we took turns relaying the unbelievable news to all our doctors, family members, and friends who had been with us through our odyssey. We were overjoyed, elated, relieved. I had never worked harder for anything in my life. I had never faced anything with higher stakes. My prior successes in life had been so minor, so unimportant. Against the odds of deadly genes, powerful political opposition, and unlikely statistical probability, Henry would survive.

For two days I lived in a state of total bliss and overwhelming gratitude.

Then I miscarried.

$\mathcal{W}$e were nearly out of time.

In the four years that had passed since we made our decision to pursue PGD, I had taken 353 injections, produced 198 eggs, and had no successful pregnancy. We had spent nearly $135,000, most of which was not covered by insurance, and far too many days apart from one another, our home, and our life. Our hopes were raised to the highest heights and crashed to the depths of despair, over and over again. There was no medical explanation for our lack of success, just bad luck, I guess. Often our best embryos had FA, while the poorest quality were FA-free/HLA matches that failed to produce a pregnancy.

We understood that our chances for Henry surviving a bone-marrow transplant would be further jeopardized if we continued to pursue PGD beyond one final attempt, our ninth, before it was too late. Drs. Gillio and Wagner had made that clear. The sicker, and therefore weaker, Henry was prior to his bone-marrow transplant, the lower his chance of survival. And the chance for his survival, even while strong, was still close to zero with a nonsibling donor. Henry *was* getting sicker. During the time that we had been pursuing PGD, his platelets had fallen from a high of 103,000 to a low of 10,000; his hemoglobin from a high of 12.2 to a low of 6.9; his absolute neutrophil count from a high of 1,900 to a low of 300. The absolute neutrophil count, which determines the extent to which you are at risk of infection, had been hovering around 400—or dangerously low—for nearly two years. His vulnerability resulted in a recent case of pneumonia and along with IV antibiotics, his treatment included two platelet and two red-cell transfusions. In other words, despite the fact that he still felt and acted like a healthy boy, Henry's bone-marrow function was in a state of collapse.

By the winter of 2000, Henry was a regular at Georgetown Hospital's Lombardi Cancer Center, where he went several times a week for blood tests that tracked the progress of his bone-marrow failure. He would bring his own Band-Aids, preferring Batman to the flesh-tone standard, and would stock the treasure box with Happy Meal toys to share with the other patients. Arriving in his ubiquitous Batman costume with fully equipped utility belt, Henry was a hit with all the doctors and nurses. Especially Suzanne.

"Can I be your girlfriend?" she asked after successfully inserting an IV into Henry's arm.

"Nope," Henry replied. "I already have one."

. . .

*J*ust about the last thing you'd want to have happen when you're a young man out on a date with an older woman is for the hostess to welcome you and hand you a set of crayons and a coloring book. Especially if she picked the *wrong* coloring book.

"This is not the one I want," explained Henry. "I want the one with the animals in it." Suzanne was impressed. "I like a man who knows what he wants," she later confided in me.

Henry was a regular at Cactus Cantina, a Mexican restaurant in our neighborhood whose delicious smell of fajitas welcomes you from blocks away. Being his favorite place to dine out, it was the destination he picked for all special occasions, and also whenever he had a craving for tortilla chips cooked just right.

Suzanne Knubel, one of Henry's nurses at Georgetown Hospital, remained unsuccessful in her many attempts to steal Henry's heart from Bella, but had safely secured a position high on his list of favorite people. Suzanne was tall, pretty, and had a friendly smile and terrific sense of humor. She also was good at finding a vein and getting a blood sample, always on the first attempt. Whenever Henry went to have his blood checked, Suzanne greeted him with a big hug. She laughed at Henry's jokes and admired his strength and good attitude. After many conversations—some to clarify that he already had a girlfriend and others about logistics—Suzanne finally secured a date with Henry, on a Saturday night, no less.

Henry watched for Suzanne's car from the wooden swing on our front porch. It was a crisp fall day and the ground was covered with leaves that crunched with each step. It was late afternoon and the sun hadn't yet set, so the pumpkins on our porch were unlit, but you could easily make out the Bat Signal we had carved the day before into Henry's pumpkin. Suzanne drove up and Henry ran down the steps and they headed out for a special Saturday night.

While they waited for the table, Henry acquired two pieces of uncooked tortilla dough for him and Suzanne to squish between their fingers.

Given the early bird nature of their timing, they were lucky and got a table by a window so they could watch the passersby. A creature of habit, Henry ordered the usual, a Sprite and some tortilla chips. He asked Suzanne to pass the salt shaker so he could meticulously salt each individual chip prior to eating it. At $1.49 for his meal, Henry was a cheap date.

They ate, talked, did word searches, and colored for the better part of an hour and went for a walk in the neighborhood when they were done.

"That was the best date I've had in months," Suzanne reported after dropping Henry off later that evening. "He is the most handsome, delightful guy I know. He really knows how to make a girl feel special."

*L*ater that month, Henry's blood tests revealed news that we had been dreading since he was first diagnosed with Fanconi. Henry's bone marrow was no longer functioning sufficiently. He would have to have his transplant soon in order to have the best chance for survival. Dr. Gillio explained that Henry could simply not afford to get sick with something like pneumonia again. It was a devastating thing to hear—a devastating realization. This time, our ninth, would be our last.

This heartbreaking development and the decision to schedule Henry's transplant for the coming summer should our final PGD attempt fail, was offset, somewhat at least, by promising news from the medical world.

Motivated by a deep desire to improve the transplant survival rate (which was just one out of every four children, most of whom did not have Henry's type of FA), Drs. John Wagner and Margaret MacMillan at University of Minnesota Children's Hospital in Minneapolis had developed a new Fanconi transplant protocol for patients like Henry who did not have HLA-matched sibling donors. This protocol was designed to address some of the deadly threats associated with bone-marrow transplants—the most serious of all being graft failure, when the new donor stem cells (the parent cells that create all blood cells) fail to "take" and grow after transplantation. In nearly every case of graft failure, the patient dies. The other major transplant complication is graft-versus-host disease (GVHD), where, due to incompatibility, the donor's bone marrow attacks the patient's organs and tissues, impairing the patient's ability to function and increasing susceptibility to infection, potentially leading to death. The greater the disparity between the HLA type of the patient and the donor, the greater the chance of GVHD. For this reason, patients who have HLA-matched sibling donors rarely get GVHD; and patients with unmatched, unrelated donors, often do. GVHD can range from an inconvenience to a deadly disease.

To avoid graft failure and foster engraftment, the new transplant protocol at the hospital in Minneapolis added the drug fludarabine to the preparative regimen—to go along with chemotherapy and total-body irradiation—to more effectively prepare the patient's body for the donor cells. The protocol also used T-cell depletion to remove the T-cells, which were believed to cause GVHD, from the donor's marrow.

The doctors believed that to have the best chance for success with the new protocol, it was critical to proceed to transplant while the patient was still relatively healthy, before there were any signs of leukemia, as signaled by abnormal clones in the bone marrow; and also before the patient became transfusion dependent. Having more than twenty blood transfusions was considered too many.

Henry had already had four blood transfusions in the past two months, and his white blood cells, red blood cells, and platelets were all far below normal levels.

Several other Fanconi patients had undergone a bone-marrow transplant under the new protocol, though it was too soon to gauge the long-term results. If we proceeded to transplant without a sibling donor, Henry would be the fifth. Yet again, we would place our faith—and Henry's life—in the hands of doctors and researchers who shared our hope but, more important, had access to the best that science could offer.

As we drove home from New York, knowing we had time for just one more chance to make this work, I thought about that morning four years earlier when Dr. Auerbach had called—the pregnancy test announcing Jack's arrival still on the table by our bed—to tell us about PGD. I thought about how relieved and grateful I had felt, and how I had carried those feelings with me all those early months, knowing that it was just a matter of time, and of science, before Henry would be OK. And now, here we were: driving home, nearly defeated, exhausted, and about to face the biggest challenge of our lives.

*T*hree months.

We could spend the time as we prepared for our ninth and final attempt worrying and stressing and feeling anxious. Or we could have the best time of our lives.

We chose door number two.

It was the easiest decision we ever made, and we started, of course, with Batman. It just so happened that at the time, Batman himself (like, the *real* Batman) was coming to Six Flags America in Bowie, Maryland, not too far from our home. When Allen told Henry, he reacted the same way I do when I hear that Bruce Springsteen is coming to town. Long before the Internet made ticket purchasing for such concerts possible, I would spend the night with friends and a cooler full of Budweiser in the parking lot at the Capital Centre in Landover, Maryland, to secure a good place in line and get tickets to the show. Thankfully for Henry, he had Allen.

Of Allen's good traits, and of those there are many, perhaps the best is his desire to anticipate and fulfill all of our needs. Allen was determined to not just get Henry tickets to the show, but to arrange a one-on-one with Batman. The morning of the show, Henry suited up in his Batman costume. He put on his mask and his utility belt, with batnunchucks and a batarang. He laced up his Batman sneakers.

"I'm ready!" he informed us, in case there was any doubt.

We got to the park, where a Six Flags customer-relations representative handed us the tickets to the live-action show and gave Henry a bright blue inflated basketball featuring the Bat signal on one side and Batman in action on the other. "Cool!" he exclaimed, dribbling the ball. The man then walked us to our seats and told us to stay put after the show was over. All of a sudden the music started blaring and the lights started flashing. It was loud. Jack, age three, started crying and covered his ears to minimize the noise of the explosions and pyrotechnics.

"I want to go home," he pleaded, suggesting that we perhaps should have heeded the signs warning of the show's unsuitability for very young children.

Henry stood on his tiptoes to get the best view. All of a sudden, Batman sped out on his Batcycle. He saved Gotham City and Vicki Vail from near-certain disaster at the hands of the Joker, and blew Henry away beyond any ten-minute encore version of Springsteen's "Rosalita" I ever heard.

After everyone left, Henry approached the stage. Batman reappeared. Henry ran over to him and said, "Hi, Batman. I'm Henry. Your cape is so cool."

Batman took a good look at Henry and said, "You look just like me," and they high-fived each other. Batman lifted Henry up and placed him on the Batcycle. Henry's feet dangled down the sides of the bike, his legs well short of the length needed to reach the pedals and take off. Big and little Batman hung out and talked about which villain was the worst (Henry was partial to the Joker) and which accessory was the coolest (the batarang, of course). Then they posed for pictures. As they said good-bye, Henry opened his arms as wide as they could go and gave Batman a huge hug. On the way home, Henry explained, "That was the best day ever. I got to see Batman. It was not a movie."

Seeing Henry's reaction to meeting Batman only increased Allen's determination to make it happen again. Destination: Florida.

Baseball fans around the country, but maybe most of all in Baltimore and DC, got caught up in Cal Ripken's streak in the mid-1990s. Cal was a star shortstop and third baseman for the Baltimore Orioles from 1981 to 2001, and was vying to break Lou "Iron Man" Gehrig's fifty-six-year-old record of playing in the most consecutive games. On September 7, 1995, about a month before Henry was born, Cal did what was once considered impossible. He played in his 2,131st consecutive game, breaking Lou Gehrig's superhuman record before a sellout crowd of 46,272 in Oriole Park at Camden Yards as the Orioles beat the California Angels 4–2. With that, Cal became the greatest iron man in baseball history.

Cal was Henry's second-favorite hero. In the summertime when we would frequent Funland, an amusement park in Rehoboth Beach, Delaware, Henry would save up the tickets he would win playing games so he could claim his prize: yet another Cal Ripken baseball card. Henry wore an Orioles baseball cap and Cal Ripken T-shirt and practiced his swing, yearning to be a professional baseball player like Cal when he grew up. Watching him whack wiffle balls from our front porch, across the street, and into the neighbor's yard, Henry's dream of becoming a professional baseball player like Cal seemed within reach. He certainly had the strength, focus, and tenacity required of an iron man.

In March, just a few weeks before I was scheduled to begin the Lupron shots for attempt number nine, we went to Florida. We set our sights on Walt Disney World, where we had a history of good times, and on Captiva, a beautiful sanctuary on Florida's west coast where we had enjoyed birds, dolphins, manatees, and shell collecting years earlier.

As it happened, the Minnesota Twins had their spring training in Fort Myers, Florida, not far from Captiva, and they were playing the Orioles while we were in town. Allen called the Twins' public-relations staff and asked if they would arrange for Henry to meet Cal Ripken.

On March 15, 2000, we arrived at the Lee County Sports Complex. It was a beautiful, sunny, and warm day—perfect for baseball. Jack and I made our way to the bleachers. Henry and Allen headed to the dugout where the meeting would take place. Henry, in his well-worn Batman T-shirt, got to swing Cal's bat, and the two of them talked for a while. When Henry and Allen joined me and Jack, I was eager to learn what they had discussed. Did Henry get the answers to big questions like "How did it feel to break Gehrig's streak?" or "How much longer would he play ball?"

"Mom," said Henry. "I met the *real* Cal Ripken! I got to hold his bat!" When I asked what they talked about, he answered, "We talked about Pokémon. I asked him which one was his favorite."

"Well, what did Cal say?" I asked.

"Charizard," he said, as if the answer was so obvious it need not be asked.

A few days later, tanned, relaxed, and happy, we returned to Washington. But we weren't done yet.

That week, I started my Lupron shots. Also that week, Allen sat the family down at the kitchen table for a very serious talk with our sons.

"Guys, listen very carefully," he boomed. "Today you are going to meet William Jefferson Clinton, the president of the United States!"

"No way!" yelled Henry. "I voted for him in school."

"Me too!" added Jack.

Allen had arranged, through our friend Peter Rundlet, who worked in the White House counsel's office, for the four of us to attend one of President Clinton's weekly radio addresses.

"Do we get to go inside the White House?" asked Henry, who, like all Washingtonians, had driven by it countless times.

"Not just the White House, but inside the Oval Office, which is probably the most important room in the whole world," replied Allen.

"Cool!" said Henry. "I'm going to wear my suit."

"Perfect! I'll wear one too," Allen said.

The boys dressed in their khaki pants and blue blazers and we headed downtown. We passed through security with a small group of people who shared the privilege of hearing the radio address live, and within minutes the kids were face-to-snout with Buddy, the president's dog, with whom they exchanged kisses for licks. When it was time for the recording, we all entered the Oval Office and were asked to keep perfectly quiet during the taping. This was easier said than done for Jack, who was merely three years old. Allen held on tight to Jack, who spent the entire time desperately trying to pull the iconic portrait of Andrew Jackson off the wall. Thankfully, the address ended before Jack was successful, and we lined up to meet the president.

"You must be Henry," the president said, when it was our turn. "I hear you are a brave little boy. It's really nice to meet you."

"Thanks!" said Henry. Not one to dwell on himself, Henry held out the toy he had been carrying and said, "This is Jake Justice. He's a Rescue Hero."

"He looks strong," said the president. "Just like you."

*F*our weeks later, my pregnancy test was negative.

*A*s we prepared to call our family and friends to tell them of our impending departure to Minneapolis, I tried to focus on the positive. The transplant would take place at the University of Minnesota Children's Hospital with a donor identified through the National Marrow Donor Program, who matched five out of six of Henry's antigens. This was the very same hospital where the first pediatric bone-marrow transplant was successfully performed, I explained again and again, and featured some of the world's most highly skilled Fanconi specialists, who had performed dozens of Fanconi transplants. We knew that this place and these doctors gave us the best possible chance that Henry could be among the first patients with his particular type of Fanconi anemia to survive an unrelated bone-marrow transplant. Once again, we would be pioneers, hoping this time that the medical breakthrough would belong to us.

"I'm so scared, but I know we have to do this now. Henry won't survive if we delay the transplant any longer," I said to my friend Karen on the phone one night, after Henry and Jack had fallen asleep. We were planning to stop at their home in Cleveland for some fun on the way to Minneapolis. "But I'd rather be doing PGD again than having a transplant that is so uncertain. I would undergo PGD nine more times—nine hundred more times—if I could."

"You did everything you could, Laurie," Karen said, her voice breaking. "I can't wait to see you and give you a hug," she added.

"Good, because I need one. A big one."

As I repeated the conversation with my family and friends that night, it was, of course, not lost on any of us that the Dickey Amendment–induced delay that interrupted Dr. Hughes's work for nearly one year had denied us the time for at least three additional PGD attempts.

One of those just might have made all the difference.

Henry's Favorite Things

- Going to Funland
- Cotton candy
- Winning stuffed animals
- Building drip castles
- Soft ice cream
- Getting buried in the sand
- Aunt Alice and Uncle Peter's beach house

10

FUNLAND

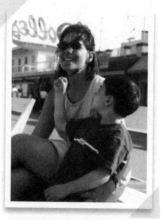

Henry tickles my chin with a magic feather on the boardwalk in Rehoboth Beach, Delaware

he Paratrooper is one of eighteen rides at Funland, an amusement park on the boardwalk in Rehoboth Beach, Delaware. The park is filled with music from a vintage carousel, mixed with the sounds of waves crashing, alarms signaling victory in Whac-A-Mole or Skee-Ball, and the laughter and cries of kids and parents overwhelmed with summertime joy. The air is filled with the salty ocean mist and the good, greasy smells of nearby popcorn and Thrasher's french fries and vinegar. Ride tickets are sold individually for 25 cents, but $10 will buy a book of 54 tickets, and nearly every adult is seen with an abundance of them.

We were barefoot in Funland. It was sunny and warm. We'd had ice cream for lunch and cotton candy for dessert. It was a few days before we were scheduled to leave for Minneapolis, but that didn't matter. Nothing mattered except one sweet fact: Henry and I were on the Paratrooper.

I had ridden the Paratrooper with friends in grade school, boyfriends in college, and Allen as a newlywed. But nothing prepared me for a ride with Henry. It all started with that look—that Henry look where his eyes sparkled extra brightly and his double dimples were tempting me to gobble him up.

And then he said, "You know, Mom, if you want to go, I'll go with you."

Of course I wanted to go. After Henry first made me a mom and I had time to think about all the stuff I wanted to do with him, one of the first things that occurred to me was I couldn't wait to take him to Funland, just like my parents had taken me when I was a kid. I couldn't wait to watch him ring the bell on the fire engine or to ride on the carousel, but most of all, I couldn't wait to ride the Paratrooper with my baby. Of course, with its height requirement, fear factor, and the threat of Fanconi anemia, it was unclear if we would ever get there.

So when he asked the question, I didn't even hesitate. We got lucky and the Paratrooper car that stopped right in front of us was Henry's favorite color: gold. The ride is like a Ferris wheel, but a lot more fun. The seats look like chairs, topped with a big umbrella. We kicked off our shoes and jumped on. The ride began to lift, going faster and faster, and we felt the wind rush through our bare toes and held each other's hands, fingers clasping fingers. As the ride peaked, we screamed as loud as we could. I looked out at the ocean and breathed and screamed and cried, and wished it would go on forever.

When we neared the bottom, we waved frantically at Allen and Jack. Every time we started our descent, we screamed as if it would never end.

When the ride was over, our cheeks were flushed and Henry's smile was as big as I'd ever seen it. We collected our shoes, and Henry and Jack were off again; darting from ride to ride, stopping for their favorites: the ball pit, the helicopter, the carousel. The tickets in my pocket slowly disappeared.

Then it was time for the games. Henry and Jack picked the game where the main prize was a Pokémon stuffed animal. The object of the game was to throw a beach ball so it would land on the rim of a red or blue bucket, which were surrounded by far too many yellow buckets. One dollar and one try later, Henry won. Arms raised and fist-pumping in victory, Henry selected Charizard, of course. Jack had greater difficulty. The first ball bounced off a bucket and landed on the boardwalk. He tried and tried, to no avail.

"You can do it, Jackie-boy!" Henry yelled while patting Jack's back.

Each loss was met with encouragement by all of us and greater frustration for Jack. Henry asked for another turn and tossed the ball right into the red bucket. Instead of choosing Pikachu or another character, he asked for Blastoise, Jack's favorite. He smiled his Henry smile and handed it to Jack. From the look on Jack's face, that was at least as good as winning it himself.

I wanted this day to last forever, and I felt my disappointment growing as the day grew dark and Allen said it was nearing time to go. But not before we stopped at Kohr Bros. for chocolate-and-vanilla-twist soft ice cream with chocolate jimmies, which Henry and Jack ate while clutching their Pokémons, sitting on a bench overlooking the Atlantic Ocean.

"Can we go to Candy Kitchen?" asked Henry.

"I want LEGO candy and wax bottles!" exclaimed Jack.

"That's what I'm going to get," Henry added.

As they ran toward the Candy Kitchen, I followed slowly behind, taking in the salt air and what was left of the warm summer sun. In my pocket I found two remaining tickets. I was about to call out to Henry, to ask him what we could get for two tickets, but at the last second, I changed my mind. Instead, I pulled out my wallet and tucked the tickets inside.

Although I knew the road we would travel would be far from easy, somehow I believed it would lead us back to Funland.

Henry's Favorite Things

- Taking pictures
  - Eskimo and butterfly kisses
    - Flying kites
  - Getting out of the hospital
- Playing Skee-Ball
  - Playdates and parties with his cousins
- Meeting President Clinton

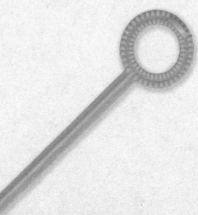

11

PLAN B

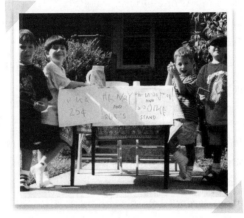

Henry, Jack, and friends—lemonade or a cookie, 25¢

s we readied ourselves for the fight of our lives, my brother, my sister, and the Ladies of the Pines, most of whom I remained close to, were planning for the superhero sendoff party of the century. On the afternoon of June 11, the day after our last Funland trip, and three days before we were leaving for Minnesota, Allen, Henry, Jack, and I walked into Temple Sinai's social hall.

I had heard that there had been a lot of planning involved, but when I pushed through the doors, I was overwhelmed. There were Batmans everywhere. Not only on the centerpieces and the cake (made especially by one of Henry's favorite people, Max, from our local ice-cream parlor) but standing along the walls, sitting on chairs, and twirling hula hoops on the dance floor. Everyone was dressed as a superhero. Our good friend Mike Rosenberg, a Washington attorney, was dressed as Batman. Michael Barr, who would later go on to work in the White House, was Robin. As soon as they saw Henry and Jack, who were themselves dressed as Batman, they ran to them, lifted them up high above their heads, and flew them around the room. The boys shrieked with excitement and the entire crowd whooped and hollered.

It was an amazing day. More than a hundred family, friends, neighbors, teachers, and doctors came dressed as superheroes as a tribute to Henry and his lifelong obsession. Of course, Bella was there. She didn't have to dress up as a princess to be one in Henry's eyes. Ari, Simon, and Jake came, as did all of Henry's cousins, aunts and uncles, grandparents, school friends, and soccer teammates. His pediatrician was there, as were his teachers Liane, Denis, and Elaine. Henry's classmates presented him with a special Batman pillowcase that they decorated and autographed. Jugglers, magicians, balloon twisters, and plate spinners entertained the kids as they posed for pictures with Batman and Robin, and celebrated the marvels of childhood.

There were gifts for Henry and big hugs all around. My favorite moment, perhaps, was when I saw my dad hand Henry a brand-new shiny silver-and-gold plastic sword. This wasn't just any sword. This was the sword that Henry would carry with him to Minneapolis, to every appointment and every procedure during his first week. I knew this was a big deal, not just for Henry, but for my dad. He is certainly not the type of guy who likes to shop. Rather, he leaves that to my mom, while he is out fishing, flying over Chesapeake Bay, or relaxing by the fire with a good book. But he had gone alone to the local toy store and picked this one out himself. I knew that it was his way of letting Henry know that regardless of the distance between them, his Papa Sy would be there with him every day, prepared to fight alongside him, and totally ready for battle.

As the evening wound to a close and the younger, wide-awake superheroes were pulled reluctantly toward the parking lot by their older, tired superhero parents, I was filled with joy and gratitude. So many people knew, understood, and loved my son. My brother Andrew came to stand beside me. We watched Henry as he stood with Jack, Bella, Ari, Simon, Jake, and his cousins Michael, Rachel, and Emma, poring through the goodies that had been hidden inside the piñata. They showed one another what they had, and made a few exchanges. He looked so happy—and perfectly healthy. I knew that what was happening on the inside made what we were about to do essential, but that didn't make it any less difficult or confusing.

Andrew put his arm around me. "You know what I think, Laurie?"

"What's that?"

"Batman should wear a *Henry* shirt."

The next morning, Henry announced that he wanted to see Bella one more time before we left for Minnesota. I called Liane and secured a date. Within hours, Bella arrived. She was dressed in a matching flowered tank top and shorts. Henry wore the new Batman Beyond T-shirt that Bella had given him at the superhero celebration the day before. Bella brought a camera with her, which she put to immediate use.

It was hot and sunny, a perfect afternoon for soccer on our front lawn. Bella and Henry teamed up against Jack and his friend Noah.

"Henry, are you the MVP on your soccer team?" Liane asked

after Henry dribbled right by Jack and Noah and scored the first of many goals.

"Yeah, because I eat a lot of food," Henry replied as he passed the ball to Bella, who dribbled it onto our neighbor's yard and into the bushes for another goal.

Jack and Noah were no match for Henry and Bella, who continued to score on each drive down the eight-foot-long field.

After the game ended, Bella went inside to get her camera. Henry put on his Batman cape for a few final shots.

I gave Liane our address in the hospital's bone-marrow-transplant unit so Bella could keep in touch. As they were preparing to leave, Bella reached into her mom's bag and pulled out a card that she had made for Henry that simply said "Luv, Bella." Inside the card were two small, soft M&M's figures, one blue, the other green. Compliments of two small pieces of velcro, they were holding hands.

"Look, Mom! Look what Bella gave me!" Henry exclaimed. He ran over to me and whispered something in my ear. It was important.

"I want to give Bella a hug," he explained.

"I think she'd like that," I whispered back.

He inched away from me and toward her. Liane saw what was going on and gently pushed Bella Henry's way.

Henry and Bella embraced. For the last time that year.

The night before we left for Minneapolis, Henry and Jack became taken with fireflies. Their interest was sudden and overwhelming, and they spent a great deal of time running around our front yard, catching one firefly after another. Each catch was a victory for my sons, though not for the bugs, many of whom gave their lives in the clumsy, innocent hands of my three- and four-year-old boys.

As I was watching them that evening from the swing on our front porch, I let my mind drift to thoughts of my own childhood, of the curiosity and wonder about the world that defines a child's dreams. When I shook myself from my reverie, I noticed that Henry had disappeared inside the house. Inside, I didn't see him on the first floor, and so I went upstairs. I slowly opened his bedroom door.

"Mom, come in quick," I heard in an insistent whisper. "Close the door."

The room was dark. And then I saw them: dozens of pinpricks of warm, yellow light, flashing and floating above Henry's head. He had carried the fireflies upstairs, one by one, cupped in his hands. Then he set them free.

"It looks like the sky," he whispered, reaching over to take my hand. He was the picture of joy, lying on his back, watching the fireflies light up his room.

It was this image of Henry that would carry me through some of the darker moments during our time in Minneapolis.

The next day, Allen, Henry, and Jack were in the car. The trunk was packed, the ignition was on, and they were waiting. I was still inside. I had turned off the lights, closed the blinds, and checked, yet again, to be sure all the appliances were unplugged. Flipping off the last light, I stepped onto the porch and began to pull the door closed. But instead, I paused. I went back inside, back upstairs, and stood in front of the door to Henry's bedroom.

HENRY.

I traced the letters on the door, the ones that had been there since he'd moved into this room, this house, our lives. I opened the door and walked in and, in the quiet, I looked around. In the closet, his costumes: Batman, Buzz Lightyear, Peter Pan, an astronaut. Under the bed: a couple of stray Batman toys, typical kid stuff. I could find nothing among his toys, his soccer cleats, or his books that justified our trip to Minneapolis. I could still see nothing in his face or smile or boundless energy that convinced me that we were doing what needed to be done. For that, I would have to study the Fanconi Anemia Research Fund's scientific updates predicting improved bone-marrow-transplant outcomes, read through our thick file of the results of his blood tests, and look at my still-bruised thighs.

We are doing the right thing. I repeated these words silently to myself as I walked back downstairs. Moving forward with Henry's bone-marrow transplant while he was still strong gave him a better chance of returning to his room and his life than waiting longer or not having a transplant at all, which on all accounts would be met with certain death. *We are doing the right thing.* I stepped onto the porch and locked the door. I had done this a million times, of course, but this time was different. I was unsure if Henry would ever step foot in the house again, or if I would ever want to. I climbed into the front seat next to Allen and turned around to Henry and Jack. "You ready for this adventure?" I asked.

"Yeah!" said Jack.

"Yeah," repeated Henry. "Off we go!"

As we began the eighteen-hour trip to Minneapolis, driving east on Calvert Street, north on Wisconsin Avenue, and out of DC, Allen took a CD from the stack: *Henry's Mix.* He slipped it into the CD player and with each new song, my mind was flooded with memories.

When Henry was three, we bought him his first boxed set, the four-volume *Nutshell Library* by Maurice Sendak, and the CD that accompanied it, Carole King's *Really Rosie.* Bedtime featured "Pierre" Henry's favorite from the set. It was also, therefore, song one on *Henry's Mix.* Allen and I would lie in Henry's bed, singing the story with Henry as he turned the pages. We would all yell, "I don't care!" as loud as we could along with Pierre and Carole. Long after we hugged him good night, exchanged butterfly kisses with a flutter of our eyelashes on one another's cheeks, and left his room,

we would hear Henry shouting, "I don't care!" until there was silence. As I recalled that wonderful bedtime ritual, on cue, Henry
and Jack yelled from the backseat: "I don't care!" Their timing was
perfect.

Tom Chapin's "Homemade Lemonade" was next. Henry's friend
Simon introduced Henry to this song on the way home from a play
date. It is an ode to the tasty superiority of the fresh squeezed,
straight-from-trees variety and the financial return associated with
one of childhood's biggest pleasures, the lemonade stand. I thought
about Henry's first lemonade stand, which he managed with the
help of Jack and his friend Jacob, and which featured a homemade
lemonade blend and fresh-from-the-oven chocolate chip cookies.
Advertised at 25 cents per cup and per cookie, the boys often got
paid more. Over the years, I have noticed that there seems to be a
correlation between the number of letters written backwards on
lemonade-stand signs and overpayment for the product. The elder
of the crowd and originator of the idea, four-year-old Henry manned
the table while Jack and Jacob ran up and down our street recruiting
customers. "Lemonade for twenty-five cents . . . or if you don't have
any money, it's free!" yelled Jack. A couple of hours later, the kids
had divided up all the money (Jack was not penalized for his social-
ist ways) and we celebrated their commercial success with ice-cream
cones at Max's.

Next: Todd Snider's "Beer Run." And yes, on a four-year-old's
mix. We easily rationalized the content by the fact that it was also a
spelling lesson, which clearly had worked. From the back seat, our
two young sons loudly sang along with Allen and me: "B double-E
double-R U-N beer run. B double-E double-R U-N beer run. All we
need is a ten and fiver, a car and key and a sober driver. B double-E
double-R U-N beer run."

Henry's CD also featured songs like "Krusty Krab Pizza" and
"Ripped Pants" featured on *SpongeBob Squarepants,* and "If I Had

a Million Dollars" by the Barenaked Ladies because Henry thought they were funny. He liked "Brick House" by the Commodores, "Out of Habit" by BR-549, and Smash Mouth's "All Star" because he could sing them while swinging his hips and dancing, which didn't work so well while he was belted into his car seat. He liked the songs written especially for him like "Henry, You're Our Super-hero" by Caron Dale, the music teacher at his preschool because . . . well, they were about him.

While Jack and Henry sang along in the backseat, up front, I struggled to make sense of our recent experience. We gave it all we had. We worked with the world's best doctors. We hoped. We believed. We were brave. We persevered. And despite all that, it didn't work.

In the end, I am left with my belief system intact. I believe in love and science. Nothing more, nothing less.

Henry's Favorite Things

- The Mall of America
- Camp Snoopy
- Rock climbing
- His shiny silver Nike sneakers
- Roller coasters
- Collecting marbles
- Sleeping in hotels

12

TAKE TWO

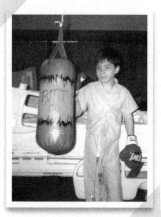

Henry, the Greatest!

*W*e had spent four years raising money for the Fanconi Anemia Research Fund, organizing bone-marrow drives that attracted hundreds of willing donors, and waiting for science to produce better drugs, better treatment protocols, improved bone-marrow-transplant success rates, and gene therapy advances. While our previous searches of the National Bone Marrow Registry initially produced eleven perfect matches to Henry, more in-depth testing showed that, of those, the best we had was merely one five-out-of-six HLA mismatched, unrelated donor.

In all likelihood, Henry's donor, like so many others on the registry, had responded to a friend's or neighbor's call for help. Ironically, in the early 1990s, long before I was pregnant with Henry, I had heard about a local woman named Allison Atlas and her need for a bone-marrow donor to cure her leukemia. When I went to get tested, a woman came up to me and said that my resemblance to Allison was striking, and that I was sure to be the perfect match. How I hoped it would be so. Sadly, I wasn't a match for Allison, who died tragically young, despite the more than 90,000 donors the organization Friends of Allison has added to the registry.

Having been told by child life specialists that it would be a good idea to talk with Henry about the purpose of our trip to Minnesota a few days before we arrived, I took the opportunity to do so when we stopped in suburban Cleveland to visit our friends Karen and Chip Chaikin along the way. I walked along as Henry, Jack, and their friend Sam Chaikin enthusiastically chased wild rabbits up and down the block. As was usually the case, Henry was the last to tire, so, when the others had had enough, he ran to my side and begged me to join him. I saw a chance to have the difficult, but necessary, talk.

I was holding his hand, searching for bunnies. "Henry," I said, "you know how we're going to Minneapolis to see the doctor?"

He nodded.

"We're going because your blood isn't working right so we are going to get you new blood."

"I know. We already talked about that," he said.

I continued, "We have to give you a bunch of medicine that might make you feel sick. Your hair might even fall out, and you are going to have to wear a mask for a long time. It will kind of be like Michael Jordan and Batman combined." I paused, trying to sense if the information I was sharing was scaring him. "All of the medicine will help the new blood find a good home in your body. It will make you all better so you can go back home and play soccer with the Dolphins and see Bella more, and the doctors a lot less." Henry listened. I stopped walking and kneeled down in front of him. "Henry, do you want to talk about anything? Do you have any questions?"

"Yeah, Mom," he said, his eyes searching the surrounding front lawns. "Where do you think that bunny went?"

When I look at photographs from our trip to Minnesota, we resembled a family heading out for spring break, having a great time. There are pictures of us at the Nike store in downtown Chicago, where Henry acquired his favorite Michael Jordan number 23 Chicago Bulls basketball jersey and sweatsuit, and in the process, ran into our own DC United soccer team. There's us having lunch and playing soccer on the shores of Lake Mendota at the University of Wisconsin. While the kids slept in the backseat, Allen and I didn't talk about the things underneath—our fears, our desperation. Instead, we talked about the things we always talked about when we took road trips: where it would be fun to stop along the way, music and musicians we liked, our family and friends, current events.

Within an hour of arriving in Minneapolis, we checked into our temporary housing, a hotel that served as overflow for the far more desirable Ronald McDonald House, which had more sick kids and families than it could hold. For years, I had been dropping extra change into the Ronald McDonald House collection box by the McDonald's cash registers in the hope that in some small way it would help those sick children get better. It was nearly impossible to fathom that my son would be one of those sick kids and that my family would benefit from the $3.49 Happy Meal that left 51 cents to help out people like us. We joined the Ronald McDonald House waiting list, hoping that someone would get better and get to go home so we could move in. At the time it didn't occur to me that sometimes families check out never to see their child again. Ever.

Henry and Jack loved staying in hotels: playing video games on the TVs, ordering room service, pushing all the buttons on the elevators. If there is a game room, forget it. They would be lost for hours. But this hotel was different. For one, we were on the ground floor, so there were no buttons to press to get to our room. There was no room service. No games on the TV or anywhere else. Our view was a parking lot. Our destination: a children's hospital.

Soon after we arrived, we put our bags in the dark and dismal room and headed out in search of some fun. I needed an immediate escape from the fear that threatened my ability to enjoy our last day together, for who knew how many weeks. As good fortune would have it, the country's biggest, brightest, busiest, noisiest, happiest place was a mere fifteen minutes away. Mall of America boasts 4.2 million square feet of retail therapy, which for me and my family was a start.

Mall of America has something for everyone. Groups of elderly people in Easy Spirit shoes walk the half-mile-plus indoor linoleum "track" on each level for exercise. Couples tie the knot in the Chapel of Love. If you can't find what you want or need in the more than 520 stores, then it probably doesn't exist. We logged eight hours in that first trip to the mall.

Jack's first choice, and therefore one of our early destinations, was the Underwater Adventures Aquarium, the world's largest underground aquarium. Jack had always been fascinated by animals, particularly those that live underwater. By that time, he had already amassed a huge collection of plastic whales, which he would line up and categorize by tooth type (baleen vs. toothed) and then again by ocean habitat. (He would later, at age seven, be invited to teach a kindergarten class on whales and dolphins.) At the aquarium, Jack darted from tank to tank, pointing out all the different types of fish. Henry chased after him. After seeing what seemed like thousands of sea creatures (4,500, if the advertisements are right), the boys arrived at the shark tank, where they had the opportunity to touch real live sharks and stingrays. As Jack explained the familial relationship between sharks and rays, Henry reached right in to touch a stingray. As Henry's hand hit the water, a shark reared its head, exposing its sharp teeth (at least this is how the boys tell it) and darted toward Henry. Jack saw it all happen, grabbed Henry, and pulled his arm out of the water. In that moment, the story about how Henry nearly got eaten by a shark—and about how Jack saved him—was born.

All that excitement made us hungry, so we headed to the Rainforest Café. With its cute animals and very full and colorful gift shop, Henry was in his element. Up until the faux lightning and thunderstorm, Jack liked it too. But with the first clap of thunder, Jack bolted out of his seat and ran as fast as he could out of the restaurant. Allen ran after him, but could not convince Jack to return. Jack waited outside, far from the thunder, while Allen informed me that Jack had accepted his offer to go to the mall's LEGO store, but refused to come back in to finish his lunch. Henry and I finished up our meals and got Jack's pizza and Allen's burger to go. Thankfully, the LEGO Imagination Center was on the same level, so we met Allen and Jack, the latter of whom was busy constructing LEGO cars to send down the ramps. Jack could have spent hours checking out the huge LEGO dinosaurs, and building and racing LEGO cars in the build-it-yourself bins. And, over time, he did.

Amazingly, right in the middle of the mall is Camp Snoopy, a seven-acre amusement park with rides, games, and junk food (also known in our family as breakfast, lunch, and dinner). We rode the Li'l Shaver roller coaster many times, raced boats, and ate ice cream. Without the Boardwalk and Atlantic Ocean, it was no competition for Funland, but it was big and loud and fun and Henry-ish, nevertheless.

I had tried to prepare myself for the moment when we had to walk into University of Minnesota's pediatric bone-marrow-transplant clinic. But when the four of us finally pushed through the wooden doors at 8 a.m. the next day, and I saw the rows of chairs filled with little kids wearing baseball caps to cover bald heads, their faces swollen from steroids and absent of smiles, I had to fight the urge to grab Henry and Jack and run back to the car. We didn't belong here in the land of the sick, where how people were doing was so obvious it was pointless to ask.

For the first five days, Allen and I had meetings: Henry's radiation therapists, his cardiologists, nuclear medicine technicians, social workers, infectious disease specialists, and, because radiation and chemo cause tooth decay, even dentists. Henry, meanwhile, endured numerous blood tests, IVs and anesthesia, a bone-marrow biopsy and aspiration, chest X-rays, an echocardiogram, kidney and liver ultrasounds, chest and sinus CAT scans, and dental X-rays. He attended a radiation-therapy consultation, radiation simulation, and a bone-marrow-transplant class, where he was offered the opportunity to play with a bald doll with a central line in his chest. Needless to say, it was no competition for the Batman figurine he brought with him.

He remained upbeat throughout it all, carrying to each appointment the sword that Papa Sy had given him. As the nurses prepared to take yet another sample of blood or insert an IV, Henry would hold that sword tight, stick it high in the air, and exclaim, "Let's get it over with and get out of here!" The nurses would burst into giggles and have to take a moment to compose themselves before inserting the needle.

Watching Henry approach these experiences—even a trip into the small, dark MRI machine—with courage and a sense of humor not only made me appreciate my son for his ability to make everything better for everyone else, but it also provided Allen and me with the strength we needed to keep signing medical release forms. And checking yet another day off the calendar. Each afternoon when the assortment of tests and procedures was over, we left the hospital and headed for something, anything, that better resembled the life we had left behind at home.

One afternoon Allen took Henry and Jack to a party in the hospital courtyard so they could meet some of the Minnesota Vikings cheerleaders and cheer for their favorite turtles during the hospital's annual Turtle Derby. I stayed in the hospital clinic to talk with the child life specialist, hoping to better understand what to expect over the next days, weeks, and months. I had spent hours and hours on the Internet searching and re-searching the Centers for Disease Control, and every other website I could find, to help prepare Henry and our family for the transplant. While there was plenty of information on the stages of the transplant process and how Henry's body would react, I still didn't know much of the critical stuff. Whether Henry could bring the blanket my mom knit for him when he was a baby into his hospital isolation room. How many weeks or months Jack would have to wait to see him. Or whether I could kiss or hold Henry.

I longed for a rule book that we could follow to guarantee that Henry would survive, but none existed.

Henry's Favorite Things

- Tae Kwon Do with Anthony, Vijay, and Mr. Kim
- The Magic Closet
- Walkie-talkies
- Wrestling with Jack
- Playing bingo
- Eating brownie batter
- Linus Van Pelt's sage advice, "Never jump into a pile of leaves with a wet sucker."

13

DAY 0

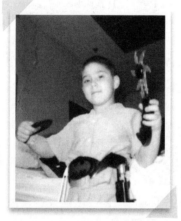

Henry, armed for action

$\mathcal{I}$t was hard being in Minneapolis, doing what we were doing, absent everything that provided comfort in our life—our friends and family, our school and jobs, our neighborhood. Our home. Everything was foreign. Initially, we spent lots of time trying to establish routines to create some semblance of normalcy. Allen and I had both secured leaves of absence from our jobs, thanks to the Family and Medical Leave Act, so we could focus every effort on getting Jack and Henry settled in Minneapolis for a four-month stay, and on Henry's recovery. My mom stayed with us for nearly the entire time. I don't know if we asked her to come or if she offered, but we needed her to be with us, and she needed to be there. She sacrificed time with my father, my sister and brother, and her other grandchildren, not because she loved us more, but because she loved us. She saw agonizing things that no grandmother should see, but Henry loved that she was there every day. Having lost her own mother as a young girl of fifteen, my mom knew to appreciate the gift of time with someone you love.

Through a medical insurance benefit that provided a generous housing allowance, we were able to rent a lovely, newly refurbished, two-bedroom apartment in the historic Calhoun Beach Club on the north shore of Lake Calhoun, one of Minnesota's 10,000 lakes. I was initially hesitant to select an apartment that was nicer and more expensive than our home in DC, and in such stark contrast to the cheerless purpose for being there, but Allen and my sister Abby, who had flown in from Washington to help us get settled, convinced me that we—and Jack in particular—would benefit from a private, comfortable, and peaceful place to live amidst the disorder of our lives. This home-away-from-home was just ten minutes from the hospital and provided easy access to parks, swimming pools, summer camp for Jack, and the peace and beauty of the lake.

In addition to my mom and Abby, so many members of our family flew to Minneapolis to be with us for welcomed stretches of time. Cousin Hannah, Aunt Jen, and Uncle Dan came, and accompanied Jack and Henry to the Children's Museum and on the Li'l Shaver roller coaster in Camp Snoopy. The boys fished at Lake Harriet with Papa Sy. They watched fireworks with cousins Emma and Sam, and Uncle Andrew and Aunt Tracey.

It helped so much having them with us, giving us all something to look forward to after finishing up Henry's medical appointments.

Each day of our first ten days in Minneapolis—when Henry was still an outpatient, and allowed to come home with us in the evenings—we checked additional medical tests off the list and learned a little more about how to balance Henry's medical needs with the fact that he was still the vibrant, funny boy he had been long before they affixed the HENRY GOLDBERG, DOB 10/25/1995 plastic band to his wrist. Despite everything, Henry still didn't think of himself as being sick. He was always just getting better. Convinced of the connection between good attitudes and good outcomes, we were determined to keep it that way. We brought our own portable DVD player to the hospital waiting and treatment rooms so that the boys could stay entertained—laughing and reciting lines from their favorite movies—right up until anesthesia was inserted into Henry's IV and he fell asleep. When he woke up, we resumed the movie or played his favorite music or walked to the vending machine armed with loads of quarters for Pringles and M&M's.

At the end of each day, we'd all gather back at the house for take-out dinners and games, or we'd go out for ice cream or to the movies. While the adults were, of course, well aware of what was at stake, none of us talked about it. What was the point? We had chosen the only real choice we had, and the only place to go was forward.

*D*ay 0.

This was how Henry's doctors referred to July 6, the day of the transplant: the day on which Henry's life would begin anew. Seven days prior to this, on June 29, Henry was admitted as an inpatient on the bone-marrow-transplant unit, and we passed the point of no return. Soon after Henry was settled into his new room, he was sent down for surgery, where a doctor inserted a central venous catheter into a large vein in Henry's chest just above his heart. This would enable doctors and nurses to administer drugs and blood products painlessly, and to withdraw hundreds of blood samples without continuously inserting needles into Henry's arms or hands.

On Day minus 6, Henry, covered in temporary Pokémon tattoos, held his blanket and smiled as he was strapped to a table and submitted to total body irradiation while listening to and singing along with his favorite Disney music, including "Heigh-Ho," "The Bare Necessities," and "I Just Can't Wait to Be King." The radiation therapist, intent on doing his very precise job, had to remind Henry to sit still and resist the urge to move to the beat of the music. Day minus 5, minus 4, minus 3, and minus 2 featured chemotherapy, which worked in concert with the radiation to destroy Henry's existing bone-marrow cells and to make room for the new marrow. Day minus 1 was a day off, and we watched movies in his room.

Allen and I, meanwhile, had enrolled in a total-immersion course in an entirely new language: cyclophosphamide, anti-thymocyte globulin, cyclosporine, heparin, and bilirubin. We went from signing consent forms for preschool field trips to the zoo to those allowing doctors to give Henry drugs that could cause nausea and vomiting, diarrhea, bleeding, liver damage, learning disabilities, infertility, and difficulty breathing. Most of these side effects are, unlike death, temporary and reversible, so we stayed focused on our ultimate goal and signed the forms.

The colorless, quiet, sanitized, isolated hospital room was a shocking difference from where we had been just two weeks earlier: school, Funland, a Dolphins soccer game, and a huge, crowded going-away superhero extravaganza. Instead of the sounds of kids laughing or screaming with delight, the only noise was the constant swishing and beeping of Henry's IV pump or the squeaking of the nurses' shoes. Instead of colorful classroom walls featuring kids' artwork or Henry's bedroom filled with soccer trophies and Pokémon posters, the hospital room walls were white and bare. Replacing the scent of fresh popcorn or cookies or cut grass was the antiseptic smell of clean. We had traded everything for almost nothing at all.

Initially the really bad times were few and far between, and we did our best to create an upbeat environment for Henry in Room 5 of Unit 4A, where he would remain for a minimum of one month in nearly total isolation—an eternity to a four-year-old. One of the first things we did was to decorate the outside of his hospital room door with pictures of Henry in his Batman costume, Henry with Jack, Henry with Bella, and a photo of our family at the beach, to show the doctors, nurses, and technicians who was living on the other side. Inside, we managed to turn Henry's room into a playroom for one, featuring a blow-up Batman chair, basketball hoop, soccer goal taped to the door, and Pokémon and Michael Jordan posters.

On one of the first days, Henry received an urgent letter. It was from our neighbors in Washington, and it read, "Hey, Batman! Calvert Street misses you and needs your help! The evil villains Catwoman and the Joker have attacked our small neighborhood. We will try our best to hold them off while you undergo your top-secret transformation. We miss you and your trusty sidekick Robin, and hope you come back soon!"

Henry also received a letter from President Clinton, who wrote: "I recently heard that you are going through a difficult time, and I want you to know I'm thinking of you. I'm impressed by the courage you've shown in facing such a tough personal challenge."

Though we were sure that Henry had what it took to win the battle, Allen decided to take one particular caution, just in case. On the second day there, Henry woke up to find a huge black-and-yellow Bat Signal painted on his window, letting his hero know that Henry could use some help.

"Wow!" Henry yelled as he carefully pulled the IV pump to which he was attached closer to the window to get a better look. "That's so cool!"

Henry took everything in stride, managing, somehow, to find the cheer in his experience. When his hair fell out, he looked in the mirror, smiled, and exclaimed, "Awesome! I look like Michael Jordan." It was far less easy for me. I had always taken solace in the fact that he looked so "normal" and healthy. That made Allen and me less scared about the idea that "underneath," he was really sick. As I looked at him rubbing his bald head in the mirror, I smiled and told him he was right. He did look cool. And handsome. But inside, I was in knots. I'd rather have avoided that truth.

Thanks to my brother Andrew and his family, though, Henry quickly had a whole complement of cool hats and bandanas to wear. And thanks to Jason, the hospital unit's child life specialist, a bright blue-and-green Franklin punching bag with the word "Pow!" printed on it hung directly above Henry's bed. As yet another day's worth of chemotherapy dripped from the IV bag through the plastic tubing and into his body, Henry donned his two bright red boxing gloves, each of which repeated "Pow!" held one fist in the air, and exclaimed Muhammad Ali–style, "I am the Greatest!"

The night before Henry's bone-marrow transplant, Day minus 1, I sat in his hospital room, unable to sleep, reading magazines that don't challenge the mind to do more than pass time. In one, I noticed Martha Stewart's calendar. Her job that day, Thursday, July 6, 2000, was to "clean freezer and refrigerator." On Henry's calendar that day, the word "transplant" appeared. Just one word with so much potential. Somewhere in the world, our donor's calendar read something equally meaningful. How I longed to spend a day, even an hour, inspecting the "use-by" dates on the food in our refrigerator.

Transplant day was considered Day 0. The hope was that by Day 21, the new bone marrow would engraft (this is when the bone marrow starts to produce new, healthy white blood cells, red blood cells and platelets), and Henry and his immune system would be on the road to recovery. Day 100—a critical milestone in the world of bone-marrow-transplant patients—seemed like a lifetime and a dream away. On Day 100, if we were among the lucky few, I figured we would go into the hospital and the doctor would remove Henry's central line, discontinue all his medicines, and send us back home. It would mean that for the first time in his life, my son would be out of grave danger.

The stem cells for Henry's transplant came compliments of a total stranger, and they arrived in Henry's room shortly after eight p.m., nearly five hours ahead of schedule. Allen was at the apartment with Jack, and so the moment belonged to me, Henry, and the stem cells of a woman I didn't even know. I wondered where she lived, if she was Jewish, if she looked like me. All I knew was that the donor was a woman, a kind and generous woman somewhere in the world, who had the ability to undo the damage that Allen's and my genes had wreaked on Henry. Earlier that morning, I had been obsessively checking the weather conditions in Minneapolis and every major city in the country, terrified that the stem cells would be diverted or destroyed on a plane. But the doctors confidently assured me that they would arrive safely, something they knew to be true because, unbeknownst to us at the time, Henry's donor was a nurse from Minnesota. She was donating her stem cells for Henry in a room just down the hall. According to the rules of the National Marrow Donor Program, both her identity and Henry's would be kept confidential, although we could—and did—communicate by letter through our donor-search coordinator. If both parties consented, we could meet following the one-year transplant anniversary.

From 8:15 to 8:30 p.m. Central Time, I lay down next to Henry in his hospital bed and held him, careful that my hug wouldn't interfere with the IV line pumping the stem cells, and a world of possibility, into him.

"Henry, remember how I told you about your new blood?"

"Yes."

"Well this is it," I told him.

"Great," he said, opening a Nestlé chocolate Wonder Ball and reaching to the bedside table. "Want to have a Pokémon battle?"

He grabbed Charizard and I grabbed Pikachu.

"Charizard, I choose you," said Henry.

"Pikachu, I choose you," I replied on cue.

"And with a fire spin, a growl, and then the powerful flame thrower, Charizard wins the battle," Henry said as the stem cells flowed into his body. From there, they had one single, critical purpose: to find their way to Henry's bone marrow, where they'd establish a home and start to produce new blood cells.

I had been told these fifteen minutes would be uneventful. They were anything but. As I lay there next to Henry, I thought, again, about the one thing that had been plaguing me since his diagnosis: We had given him Fanconi anemia. While I never *blamed* myself or Allen, or either of our mothers, who had passed it on to us, I believed that PGD would enable us to take it away. We tried everything to make that possible. But at the moment of the transplant, as I held my son while a stranger's stem cells dripped slowly into his body, I felt at peace. For the first time since I had heard the words "Fanconi anemia," I relinquished control, accepting that it was now out of my and Allen's hands. I held Henry tightly to me, believing it would all work out. Knowing that Henry could survive.

Henry's Favorite Things

- Cracking open the Batman piñata each year at his birthday party
- Joker's Child in Fair Lawn, New Jersey
- Vending machines stocked with Pringles and Skittles
- Electric blankets
- The Glen Echo (Maryland) carousel
- Hitting Wiffle balls off our front porch
- Going to kindergarten

14

A New Beginning

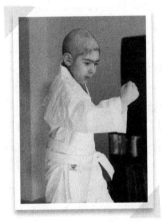

Henry shows perfect form

"I thought the stem cells were going to arrive later tonight," Allen said when he came into Henry's room and found us sitting on Henry's bed, the transplant behind us. "I can't believe I missed it."

"I'm sorry," I said. I knew that he was going to be disappointed. I stood to hug him. "It only took fifteen minutes."

Allen took a seat on the edge of Henry's bed. "Hey, Hen, do you feel any different? Are you craving food other than Pringles?"

Allen asked, wondering aloud if Henry might already have adopted some of his donor's tastes. Thankfully, along with the stem cells for the transplant, a nurse had come equipped with a Polaroid camera to document the occasion. Allen flipped through the images: Henry with the stem cells, Mom and Henry with the stem cells, Henry eating his chocolate Wonder Ball while the stem cells flowed through his IV, Mom and Henry after it was over. The stem cells didn't look any different from the liquids in the bags already hanging on Henry's growing IV tree—morphine, insulin, methylprednisone, GCSF, cyclosporine—pumping into his central line in an around-the-clock, well-orchestrated attempt to save his life.

We had been told by Henry's doctors that the most unpleasant side effects of the radiation and chemotherapy would begin around Day 2 and last until Day 15 or so. Although I had originally anticipated that Day 0 through Day 21 would just be about surviving and flipping the pages of the calendar on the wall, they were, at first, about a whole lot more. Our main job was to help Henry through the side effects, and to wait and hope for a sign that the transplant had worked. Every morning a nurse would come and take a blood sample from his catheter to see if his bone marrow was producing blood cells. Rising blood counts were the best, and only, sign that the transplant was working.

The things that Henry could and couldn't do during his transplant recovery changed over time. Because the chemotherapy and radiation had almost fully disabled his immune system, during the beginning stages, his body was unable to fight infection. This meant that he could have little to no direct contact with the outside world. Although there had been some progress in treating infections, prevention remained the best strategy. Henry was taking numerous intravenous antibiotics throughout the day and night to protect him against viral, bacterial, and fungal infections. He had to brush his teeth and the inside of his mouth with a special pink sponge toothbrush five times a day, and get frequent sponge baths and bandage changes to prevent infection around his main catheter. I became accustomed to washing my hands every time I entered Henry's hospital room or touched food, a toy, my hair, or anything else before touching him. After a week, my hands were red and raw. I knew to wear the purple, sterile gloves when I helped Henry to the bathroom because it was dangerous for me to touch his urine, post-chemotherapy. I knew that right after Henry threw up and had finally fallen back to sleep was the best time to race down the hall to the bathroom, since using Henry's was prohibited. I knew that the night nurse would come in around six in the morning to give me a copy of Henry's daily blood count so I could search for any signs of hope.

For the first few weeks, only Allen, my mom, and I could visit Henry, and one of us was always there with him, right next to his bed, in his eight-by-ten room, every hour of the day. Allen and I switched off days with Henry while the other spent the day with Jack. We were horrified when anyone other than Henry's doctors or nurses asked to gain entrance to Henry's room, such as the hospital volunteers who wanted to know if we wanted a break to take a walk or have a meal. Although I put on a brave face for Henry, and for others, I was terrified. I knew he was in pain. Watching a grimace conquer his smile, seeing him lose his hair and be tethered to a wall of machines was more chilling than what I had been imagining since we made the decision to come to Minneapolis.

Between Day 6 and Day 10, any fear I may have held that perhaps the radiation and chemotherapy weren't working were dismissed as he suffered their side effects. Henry threw up almost daily, and developed mouth sores that looked more painful than he was willing to admit. Day 6 brought a real scare in the midst of all the others: Henry ran a fever of 102.7, indicating an infection (to the doctors) and that Henry was going to die (to me). But several hours and three antibiotics later, the fever was down and things went back to normal to the extent that anything in a pediatric bone-marrow-transplant ward is normal.

$\mathcal{H}$enry's pain eventually worsened. The only thing we could do was give him morphine, which meant that all he did was sleep. He needed this to heal, but as I sat beside him, holding his hand, watching him sleep, my heart nearly broke. His joking, laughing, and stamina were gone, replaced by an eerie silence interrupted only by his slow, steady breath and the beep, beep, beep of the monitors that surrounded him. He had always seemed so big and strong, and now he was tiny and vulnerable. I'd say the same exact thing about myself.

Allen and I each took twenty-four-hour, two p.m. to two p.m. shifts, eating meals my mom would drop off for us. At night, we rested—I wouldn't say we got much sleep—on a twin bed the hospital had provided for us. Many days, Allen and I would see each other for only a few minutes as we exchanged medical updates, car keys, and a quick kiss during our shift change.

Because we were in a small room closed off from the world, there was no one to talk to about how scared and worn out I was. Unwilling to share my fears with Henry or to have him hear me talk about them on the phone, I kept those feelings to myself. But sometimes, rarely, I allowed myself the space to feel the weight of it all. Sometimes, in the quiet darkness in the middle of the night, I would curl up at the base of Henry's hospital bed and just gaze at my boy lost in a morphine-induced slumber. Because he was asleep, neither his smile nor his cheerful voice could distract me from his desperate medical situation. Mesmerized by the perfectly timed beat of Henry's medical pump, pushing fluids into and out of his body, my tears would flow unabated by any will or need to hide them. Raw, vulnerable, and terrified, I wondered how my life had led to this place.

And how in the world we'd make it out alive.

*G*iven our isolation, we longed for contact from the outside world and spent a lot of time waiting for the moment the mail arrived. I think Henry broke the hospital record, receiving twenty-four packages one day, some containing Batman stickers, some with action figures, others with books or puzzles or games. All made him happy.

One even contained a celestial chart depicting a star that our friend Evan had purchased and named "Batman" in Henry's honor. But the coolest of them all was a book titled *Henry Goldberg and Batman Solve the Case of the Stolen Robot*. Some ingenious friends, Harriet and Larry Berlin, had found a company that creates personalized books and knew that it was just the thing that Henry needed to break the tedium that had set in as he entered his fourth week of complete isolation in his hospital room. "Henry Goldberg looked out the taxicab window. He was very excited. All around him were the skyscrapers of Gotham City. Gotham was even bigger than he had imagined back at home in Washington." I read on, and the white walls of Henry's hospital room and the constant beeping from the IV stand cluttered with noisy medical devices faded away, and we escaped to a world that was far more fun and exciting than the one that Fanconi anemia required that we live in.

When things started to get harder, Allen and I—and Henry especially—were thrilled to find that we had gotten lucky. It just so happened that Henry's room was equipped with a Magic Closet.

Batman and Pokémon of all shapes and sizes lived inside. So did toys and gifts sent from people all over the country who loved Henry. When he threw up or got a fever or had to make it through the twenty-eighth dose of medication of the day, or a third or fourth or fifth attempt to insert an IV into the bruised vein on his arm, hand, or foot, the Magic Closet delivered.

"Holding a Pokémon helps, especially the water type," Henry carefully explained to a nurse one day. "But the Magic Closet *really* helps."

This short-term solution became a way of life. It was our way of acknowledging the hardship and trying, in the smallest way, to compensate Henry and Jack for it, one challenge at a time, and to provide incentives to keep going. Call it war reparations. Call it positive reinforcement. Whatever.

Months later, I would receive a call from a woman named Rachel Grossman, whose son Jacob was scheduled to have a bone-marrow transplant at the same hospital, asking for advice. When I finished explaining what to expect, where to live, where to eat, and what to ask the doctors, Henry asked to speak with her. He provided what he thought was the most essential advice on bone-marrow transplants, and that was to ensure that they got a room with a Magic Closet.

Jack had an especially hard time understanding why he and Henry had to be apart from each other for more than one month when Henry was most vulnerable to infection.

"That's not a good plan, Mom," Jack explained to me one night as I tucked him in, in his new Minneapolis bedroom. "Brothers stay together."

"I know," I said. "But maybe we can think of some other ways you guys can be together without being in the same room."

"Like what?" he asked.

"Like, what if you send him some pictures and write him notes," I suggested, hoping he wouldn't pick up on the fact that given that they were three and four, neither he nor Henry could read or write. He thought it was a good idea, and went to work on drawing pictures for Henry. They mostly had to settle on waving to each other, though. Henry would look out from his hospital room at Jack, who stood on his tiptoes at the top of the slide at the hospital playground in the courtyard below.

"I see him, Mom!" Jack would yell, pointing to one of the hundreds of windows in the hospital. "He's right there!"

We were determined to keep Jack happy and distracted from his separation from Henry and our general hardship. Each day Allen, my mom, or I took him to and from day camp, and then on daily outings to one of the lakes, a local bookstore, or one of the many local museums or animal habitats. On my days with Jack, I would leave the hospital at two p.m., grab the biggest cup of coffee I could in the hospital lobby to chase away my exhaustion, shift my state of mind, and run out the front door for a day of activities. Jack loved identifying the species of fish at Underwater Adventures Aquarium, riding the monorail or visiting the butterfly pavilion at the Minnesota Zoo, and manipulating the huge metal dinosaurs at the Science Museum of Minnesota. To this day, Jack's favorite thing to do is to go to zoos and museums to feed his nearly insatiable desire to expand his mind. We often visited Wild Rumpus, a local bookstore that leaves you thinking, "So many books, so little time." Housing thousands of children's books along with real chickens, rabbits, fish, birds, cats, and even a tarantula, Wild Rumpus may well have been Jack's favorite spot in Minneapolis. By the time we left town, we had acquired every book in the Magic School Bus, Magic Tree House, and Secrets of Droon series, and left empty store shelves that at one time were filled with books on sharks, whales, and dinosaurs.

Although he seemed fine, Jack occasionally reminded us that he knew what was going on. One morning I awoke around six thirty to find him crawling into my bed.

"Mom, I had a nightmare."

Gathering him into my arms, I asked him to tell me all about it.

"Henry was in a volcano and smoke was coming out. And there were evil people there." He sounded scared and, my heart breaking, I asked what happened next. He thought about it and continued, "Then Henry jumped out and flew away like Batman."

*I*n the evenings of the afternoons I spent with Jack, I'd come home to a dinner prepared by my mom, or our friend Steven Goldstein, a Minneapolis resident and Culinary Institute of America graduate who clearly knew his stuff. After reading Jack to sleep, I would leave him with my mom and walk downstairs to the gym in our building, where I would ride the stationary bicycle in a vain attempt to retain my health and sanity. Any illness, however slight, would banish me from Henry's room, which was a strong incentive to keep pedaling, despite my utter exhaustion. I would return to the apartment to soak in the bathtub and try to remind myself that things would get better. Eventually I fell asleep with the phone next to my pillow in case Allen called. In the morning, I would wake up early and call Allen to check on Henry's daily blood counts, make Jack breakfast, and drive him to summer camp. On my way back home, I would drive to the shores of Lake Calhoun, take my Rollerblades out of the trunk of the car, clip my Walkman to my shorts, and do laps around the lake, listening to Steve Earle's "Transcendental Blues" on repeat.

The life I was living was so different from the one I had expected. My sorrow, fear, loneliness, and exhaustion threatened to crush me, but I remained fiercely determined to be a good mother and give my kids the best life I could. Allen's insistent optimism was fueled by mankind's remarkable scientific achievements that made the seemingly impossible possible. In our short lifetime, we put a man on the moon, drafted a map of the human genome, and experienced the advent of the Internet. If we could do that, Allen reasoned, surely Henry's doctors could save his life. Though our perspectives varied, we agreed on the importance of making every day matter. Just in case.

At seven a.m. on Day 11, the monotony of isolation, fear, and morphine-induced quiet was interrupted by the miracle of an absolute neutrophil count of 100—a sign that the new marrow was starting to produce blood cells. I knew from the doctors and from following friends' transplants that this number could be lower tomorrow (not so good) or higher tomorrow (great!), and the same held true for the days to come. In our new world, with every piece of good news, there was often bad. Within minutes of learning that Henry's new bone marrow was on its way in, we also learned that his bilirubin count (a liver enzyme) was eight times what it should be. We spent hours worrying about the possibility of veno-occlusive disease—a serious liver disease and occasional transplant complication—before it was ruled out. No matter how much practice we'd had, these ups and downs never got any easier.

Four weeks into his recovery, Henry's blood counts were showing a consistent increase. This meant that he was better equipped to fight off infection and that Jack could visit him in the hospital. Before entering Henry's room, Jack stopped at the cleansing station outside Henry's door. He scrubbed his hands and arms for the length of a barely audible rendition of "Happy Birthday," which was supposedly enough time to sanitize them, and we placed a protective mask over his mouth and nose to ensure that he did not expose Henry to any germs he wasn't strong enough to fight. At three, Jack's face was small, and once he had his mask on, only his eyes showed. They were sparkly. He left his dirty, light-up Power Ranger sneakers outside the door to Henry's hospital room, and eagerly entered.

"Hi, Henry!" said Jack.

"Hello to you," Henry responded enthusiastically. "Want to watch a movie?"

And with that, the Dynamic Duo was reunited after nearly four weeks apart. For the rest of the afternoon, and long into the evening, Jack lay in the chair next to Henry's bed and they watched Pokémon movie after Pokémon movie. Eventually Henry fell asleep and Jack took out his Game Boy and played games, content to be with his big brother.

Jack's quiet and calm in the face of adversity brought wisdom and a sense of peace to our family, and made him someone Henry wanted to be around, regardless of how he was feeling. While most three-year-olds have a hard time sitting still or keeping quiet, Jack was content to spend that night—like so many other days and nights—hanging with Henry, even if that meant quietly waiting beside his bed until Henry was ready to wake up.

During these periods of isolation, Jack also seemed to sense his role as Henry's conduit to the outside world. Whenever he ventured out, he often wanted to get something to bring back to Henry. Sometimes it was a map of the local zoo, so Jack could explain to Henry where every animal was, what species or genus it was from, and whether it had any unique characteristics. Other times it was a chocolate croissant or Skittles or some other longed-for food. Jack never made Henry feel as if he was missing out on anything. In fact, I think Jack looked at wherever Henry was as the place to be, and often he couldn't wait to get back there. As long as they had each other—and plenty of movies, cartoons, Batman and Pokémon figures—they were more than content.

*E*lated.

That is definitely the best word I can use to describe how I felt on Day 34, when Henry was first released from the hospital. Actually, it would be more accurate if I could take the word, blow it up 1,000 times, and surround it with bright flashing lights, Vegas-style.

It was a huge milestone because it meant that his bone marrow was functioning and his immune system was strong enough to leave the safety of the hospital room. And more important, it was a major sign to us that his doctors had faith that he would survive.

There had been a lot of small, significant steps leading up to this day, as Henry was slowly emerging from being a very sick boy to being himself. He got out of bed, and we cheered. Then he was strong enough to stand. Then he was allowed out of his room and onto the transplant floor; first in a wheelchair and then walking on his own. He'd wear a protective face mask and trail a very cluttered IV pole behind him—a tangle of pumps, tubes, and bags of medications flowing into his body. On the first day he was allowed outside, Allen sat with him on an overcast day in the hospital courtyard and later told me that for the first time in weeks he thought to himself: *Henry is going to make it home.* I was so happy that Allen had the honor of being the first to see Henry reentering the outside world. Now we each had our own special firsts.

On the day itself—Day 34—I walked into Henry's room, grabbed blue and orange markers, and wrote on the dry-wipe board on the wall, usually crowded with daily medical instructions: HENRY IS GO-ING HOME! We then carefully set Henry, who was still weak from the medication and the number of days he had spent lying in bed, into a red plastic Radio Flyer wagon.

"I can do it all by myself," said Jack, as he pulled the wagon, and Henry, out of his room, down the hall, into the elevator, across the lobby, and out of the hospital. That's what sidekicks and best friends do.

The apartment in Minneapolis seemed so much more like home once Henry was back with us. We were all so excited, as it was the first time in more than a month that we would all spend the night in the same place. When we arrived at our apartment, Henry had a package waiting for him from our friend Ashley Stringer from back

home. He had sent Henry a huge gold trophy he had won in a soccer tournament and which he wanted Henry to have. Henry loved
it. He held it up in the air with a huge smile and a bald head. He
was a champion.

We couldn't return to DC for at least another two months because Henry had to continue to see his doctors daily, but at least we
were all back together. I had attended an hour-long discharge class
at the hospital a couple of days before Henry was ready to leave the
inpatient transplant unit. By that time, I was proficient at changing
the sterile bandage that protected his catheter site. My prior experience had merely involved Neosporin and Band-Aids over scraped
knees. To change Henry's bandage required wearing a mask and
sterile rubber gloves and unfolding a disposable cloth on which I
laid out alcohol swabs, Betadine antiseptic swabs, gauze pads, adhesive tape, adhesive remover, and a sterile Primapore bandage.
The first time I saw this display of materials and observed the bone-
marrow-transplant unit nurse doing the "sterile bandage change,"
I hearkened back to the day we brought Henry home from the hospital when he was born. I had watched my mom change his diaper
and his undershirt and thought to myself, "I'll never be able to do
that on my own."

The day before we left the hospital, Henry had a nurse who
tended to him twenty-four hours a day; the day we left, he had a
mom who did. When we arrived at our apartment in Minnesota, a
nurse met us with a week's worth of medical supplies: dozens of
vials of heparin and saline; 10cc and 5cc syringes; catheter valves
and replacement caps; cannula clamps; a case of alcohol swabs, Betadine swabs, and Primapore bandages; a pump to deliver Henry's
IV nutrition; tubing for the pump; a cooler with three bags of his
IV nutrition (more would be sent after the following day's blood
test revealed other nutritional deficiencies). This filled four large
cardboard boxes and, when added to the supply of cyclosporine,

fluconazole, acyclovir, Bactrim, and nystatin that Henry took by mouth a total of seventeen doses daily, it looked like more than my background in public relations and community development could handle. I listened intently and wrote furiously as the nurse showed me how to program Henry's pump so it would administer the nourishment he needed through the night to grow stronger. Back at the hospital, each of these things seemed like one more thing that would help Henry get better. In our apartment, each seemed like one more opportunity I had to mistakenly kill him.

There were so many things to learn and do, it was easy to avoid finding time to figure out what to be scared about or what to talk about with Allen or my mom or anyone else. By the time I hooked up one antibiotic, it was time to take the next medication out of the refrigerator or to give Henry a sponge bath or to try to convince him to eat something—anything. Before I could complete whatever I was trying to do, the pump would beep, signaling the end of one medication and the start of another. With more than eighteen different medications a day, this routine continued around the clock. It was rare that I slept more than thirty minutes at a time.

Once Henry was discharged from the hospital, one of the first things he asked was if he could get a karate instructor so he could begin working on his white-belt basics. After seeing Batman put his karate skills to masterful use, Henry wanted to give it a try. Plus, he was incredibly determined to get strong. The strength of the chemotherapy was apparent from Henry's bald head, but it was powerless against his endless desire to master new skills, build his strength, and defeat Fanconi anemia. Henry and his martial arts instructor, Anthony, who, to Henry's enormous delight, had played a Blue Power Ranger in the *Power Rangers* television series, worked together several times a week.

After his lesson one afternoon, Henry announced, "I'm ready to show you my form. It's called the Young Han." Anthony nodded to Henry, who was dressed immaculately in his white karate uniform cinched with his white belt. They each stood with their feet together and took a bow.

Anthony yelled, "Ready stance! Fighting stance!"

Henry followed Anthony's commands and together they yelled, "Hi Ya!"

Anthony continued: "Step. Punch. Two kicks. Step. Knife hand. Snap punch. Turn. Step. Punch. Step. Knife hand. Two kicks. Snap punch. Turn." Henry methodically did every move with Anthony and at the end exclaimed, "Hi Ya!" just before he took his final bow. Jack, my mom, Allen, and I gave him a standing ovation.

I was thrilled one day, not long afterward, to get a call from my friend Val Syme.

"How's it going?" she asked.

"He's back with us," I said, unsure, exactly, of how to answer that still-unanswerable question.

"Great. I'm coming to visit you," she said from her cell phone in New York.

"That's crazy!" I told her. "You have no idea how insane it is here." A few days later, Allen picked Val up from the Minneapolis airport and that night, my mom insisted that she stay at the apartment with the kids while Allen, Val, Steven Goldstein, and I go out to dinner. Val is loud and funny and reminds me a lot of myself when I'm not scared and in desperate medical straits. Sharing tales of the life of a single New Yorker over food that did not come delivered in a paper bag, she made me laugh out loud, which felt so good and so hopeful, and like something I hadn't done in a very long time.

When we returned to the apartment, relaxed and full, Val turned to my mom. "Nana, what did you have for dinner?" she asked.

My mom confessed to not have eaten anything. Val looked at her in disbelief, and then grabbed my mother's hand.

"You're coming with me." At ten p.m. Val was out with my mom, sharing her second dinner of the evening.

That dinner was the very least of everything that my mom deserved. She did so many things that made our life easier while we were in Minneapolis—and even when we weren't—that it is impossible for me to adequately describe, and even harder for me to properly thank her. She made a pot of hot coffee each morning. She stocked our refrigerator with vegetarian food for me, dairy-free food for Allen, and everything that Jack or Henry even mentioned that they liked to eat. She bought books for Jack; and Pokémon and Batman figures for Henry. She took phone messages and returned calls. She helped me negotiate with the insurance company. She encouraged me and Allen to take a walk or Rollerblade around the lake so we could share some quiet time.

She held us all together.

$\mathcal{D}$r. Wagner, Henry's transplant specialist, was also the doctor for the other PGD pioneering family, the Nashes. They had long since given up waiting for us and had found other doctors in Chicago, who gave them a chance to save their daughter, Molly, through PGD. While we were still in Minneapolis, the Nashes arrived with Molly and new baby Adam, conceived through IVF and PGD. The stem cells from Adam's umbilical cord enabled Molly to sail through her transplant. I was genuinely happy for them, but it was hard to have a front-row seat to watch PGD fulfill its promise.

While they recovered from their transplants, Henry and Molly slipped out of their isolation rooms so we could take a group photo of the two families. We had suffered the same diagnosis, held on to the same dream, but no longer shared the same fate. It was hard to sort out the tangle of feelings. I felt vindicated by the success of their PGD, victimized by our own failure, and overwhelmed with fear for Henry's life. I was certain that pursuing PGD over and over again had been absolutely the right thing to do. Molly Nash was living proof of this.

The media surrounding the Nashes' story was phenomenal. It spawned articles focusing on the miracle of science as well as warnings about eugenics and the creation of life for spare parts. Online discussions raged about embryo destruction and murder. While the media didn't address what would happen if we turned back the hands of time and took away the science, as Henry was hospitalized with yet another serious infection, we knew what could happen without PGD.

We spent the next seventy-five days in Minneapolis doing our best to protect Henry from viruses, germs, and other things that would threaten his fragile condition. We bought air purifiers for each room, a top-of-the-line HEPA-filtered vacuum cleaner, and what seemed like every antibacterial cleansing product in the Twin Cities area. My mom, Allen, and I scrubbed our apartment until our hands were raw. We visited the bone-marrow-transplant clinic every day, where Henry and Jack spent hours watching DVDs on their portable player or playing with their Game Boys, eating vending-machine food, waiting for results, transfusions, good news. Every day while we were out, my mom vacuumed and cleaned our apartment since Henry couldn't be around the dust. We washed Henry's clothes and sheets separately in hot water; always left the top of the washing machine open when it wasn't in use to minimize the chance of mildew; scrubbed the bathtub after each use; never left wet towels out; didn't bring home any fresh fruits or vegetables; used paper towels instead of sponges or kitchen towels; never shared food or drinks with Henry; avoided public places and sunshine; avoided fresh paint and construction sites; carried a portable potty and urinal in case Henry needed it on the ten-minute drive to and from the clinic; and hoped things would get easier.

Most of my time was spent in the apartment doing all of Henry's nursing. I would flush his IV lines with saline, program his pump, and hook him up to a medication that took one hour to flow. After a few minutes, I would get the next medication out of the refrigerator to cool to room temperature, line up all the vials of saline to flush his lines, change his bandages, and put new batteries in his pump. It was a twenty-four-hour-a-day responsibility with no room for error. When there was a break, I played games with Henry and Jack. Allen and my mom did all the errands related to meals, restocking the Magic Closet (which miraculously relocated to our apartment), doing the laundry, changing Henry's bedding every day—everything that keeps most of us busy most days without all the medical challenges.

I was depleted and scared. One mistake with Henry's medications or getting air in his lines, anything, could be deadly (or at least it felt that way). We were also severely sleep-deprived. At the same time, we were trying desperately to enjoy the time we had together, which we did not take for granted. Our ultimate goal, after getting Henry better, was to be present in every day, in every good moment. We never knew when something might go wrong, leading Henry to be readmitted, or worse, develop a deadly complication. Allen and I each felt a constant, endless pull between being drained and scared and fiercely determined to smile, laugh, have fun, and energize the kids.

Allen's parents, who were home in the Washington suburbs seeking treatment for Allen's mother's cancer, bought Henry and Jack a battery-operated ride-on car, which the boys rode on the secluded patio outside our apartment in the evening when no one else was out. Henry wore his mask and drove the car with Jack riding on the back. They were so happy to be back together after such a long absence. We were inventive, figuring out lots of fun things to do without coming into contact with other people. Thanks to some friends from Allen's office, the boys had battery-operated small plastic boats that they could race and crash into one another in the fountain on our patio. We frequented drive-through McDonald's and visited all the Snoopys on display outdoors throughout St. Paul in a tribute to the city's late favorite son, Charles Schulz.

We bought walkie-talkies so Jack could call out to the car and let Henry know what new Batman or Pokémon figures were available in the toy aisle at Target. "Henry, are you there? Are you there?"

"I'm here, Jack. Please tell me you found an Onyx."

"I'm still looking," Jack said, although, because he had forgotten to push the button when he spoke, the only thing Henry heard was "king."

"King? What are you talking about? Jackie, push the button when you talk!"

Jack tried to juggle the walkie-talkie and the Pokémon figures in his hands as everything fell to the floor. I offered to push the button and hold the equipment to his ear so he could deliver the news.

"They have a Pikachu on a surfboard. It's really cool!" relayed Jack, standing starry-eyed before the tall shelves. "Mom said I can get one."

"I definitely want that too," Henry confirmed. "But do they have an Onyx? I need an Onyx. It's *really* strong."

"Mom, is there Onyx?" Jack asked me as he put down the walkie-talkie and wandered to the superhero toys one aisle over. I got on the walkie-talkie to reassure Henry that we had some great finds and we'd be right out.

Our hunt for the Onyx was unsuccessful, but this would not be our last mission.

. . .

The riskiest thing we did was when Allen arranged for the four of us to go to the Mall of America's Warner Bros. store (the distributor of all things Batman and Pokémon) early in the morning before it was open to the public, so Henry and Jack could have a private shopping extravaganza. Allen had called the manager and explained the situation. I think it took her about one millisecond to get on board and agree to what he asked.

As we prepared to go, I heard the beep on the portable IV pump signaling the end of Henry's latest dose of antibiotics, and I disconnected his medication from his central IV line. Henry, still bald from chemotherapy, was singing a song, which he had himself composed, just right for the occasion: *"I have a wish that came true. And I'm getting to go to the Batman Store. It's true. I have a wish, that wish came true. The wish, wish, wish came true."*

Jack smiled and chimed in, *"I'm gonna choose. Hmmm. I'm going to get a Batman."* Just before we left our apartment, Henry put on his protective face mask to mitigate the risk of dangerous germs. The two boys sang and danced all the way to the car, then from the car into the mall and up to the closed metal door blocking their passage into paradise. The mall was quiet but for their Batman-related chatter. All of a sudden, the door clanked and slowly rose. Henry and Jack ducked under, ran inside, and darted from one display to another. After weighing all the options and making some hard choices, they each picked a few special things. We paid for everything and left without seeing another customer. Jack and Henry tore the wrapping off their new toys, and the Pokémon battles started before we even left the parking garage.

We understood that for the period of one year, we would be stuck in a complicated maze of difficult options, having to constantly weigh the risks associated with exposure to germs with Henry's and Jack's emotional wellbeing. We would use our well-tested "no regrets" policy as a guide—decide what we were comfortable doing, do it, don't look back, and hope like hell that we got it right.

On the September day that all of Henry's and Jack's friends started preschool back in Washington, Henry was under anesthesia in the operating room at University of Minnesota Children's Hospital.

Here, doctors extracted a small piece of his hip bone and a sample of bone marrow to get a close look at whether the donor's cells had made their way to Henry's marrow and were starting to produce new, healthy cells. Later that day as Henry recovered in his hospital room, we learned that his bone marrow was filled with 100 percent donor cells, which was incredibly promising news. It indicated that we had benefited from the new protocol and managed to avoid graft failure, a major complication that had previously taken so many young lives. We were joyful and relieved.

Hours later, however, we were deeply saddened. While standing in the hallway outside Henry's room in Unit 4A, Allen and I heard the news that a little boy with Fanconi anemia who had been fighting for his life in that same unit long before we arrived and well after Henry was originally discharged to outpatient status, took his last breath. We had not known the family, but earlier that day had seen them in the hallway, quietly talking to the doctors, holding on to one another. My heart ached for his family and friends who suffered through his diagnosis, cherished every day of his life, celebrated the success of his engraftment, worried through the sudden loss of his bone marrow graft six months post-transplant, and now mourned his premature, tragic death. It wasn't lost on me that they, too, had celebrated victories like ours that day.

Our lives became defined by the same endless routine. Each day began with a blood test to determine whether Henry needed a blood transfusion. The kids would be well into their first movie when, an hour or so later, we'd get the results, which more often than not indicated that he did. We would wait another hour or more for the blood product to arrive and then spend hours waiting for the transfusion to run its course. Often we would arrive mid-morning and leave for our apartment in the late afternoon. With three or more movies behind them and some Pringles, M&M's, and hot chocolate in their bellies, the kids were doing fine, and they'd happily walk out of the clinic, excited to get back to the apartment. Allen and I, on the other hand, were exhausted and the long and uncertain road to recovery was an everyday reminder of the consequences of our failure with PGD.

But we felt lucky. Because we *were* lucky. Despite living in a world where from time to time we had to clear the hallway as the body of a small child hidden under a drape was transported from the transplant unit to the mortuary, we were doing relatively well. Allen and I had two beautiful, resilient children. We had a life filled with good people who loved us, and good values. I felt cared-for and connected to a wonderful community and an amazing husband. We had the best doctors in the world, who were doing everything they could to save our son.

When we first arrived in Minneapolis, Henry's doctors told us that if everything went as planned, we would be able to return home to Washington in October, sometime around Day 100. The last month of our stay in Minneapolis, therefore, was marked with a manic pull between the nearness of our planned departure date and the reality that Henry was still being admitted to and released from the hospital with fevers and infections. He was also still dependent on blood transfusions. As he spent yet another day in the hospital, he had to undergo blood cultures, skin biopsies, and other tests to determine the cause of his complications and identify the most effective treatment plan. With each blood draw, transfusion, or other medical treatment, Henry would grin and exclaim "Let's just do it!" so he could get out of the hospital and get back to living his life. The tests were often inconclusive, but his fever would dissipate, his energy would increase, and we'd be sent back to the apartment a little less confident and a little more scared. I willed him to get better, and every time he overcame another challenge and got good results on the latest test, I'd fall asleep dreaming about the day we could return home. My desire to go home was so strong that when I woke up the following morning, I swore I could taste the fajitas at our neighborhood favorite, Cactus Cantina.

*M*ore than four months and a lifetime after departing for Minneapolis, on October 23, 2000, Day 100 arrived. When the clock struck midnight that day, there were no fireworks. Instead, it started and ended much like almost every other day since we'd arrived in Minneapolis. Henry took about seventeen doses of antibiotics, had spent the previous night on an intravenous nutrition pump since he had not yet regained his appetite, and suffered with chronic and painful diarrhea. We remained isolated from other people and spent hours in the bone-marrow-transplant clinic getting platelets and red-blood-cell transfusions and other supportive therapies. We arrived that day, just like we had every other day, with enough provisions to guarantee a good time even if we were confined to a small, sparsely appointed treatment room lacking the benefits of basic cable or anything else to distract the kids from how far away from anything fun we were. We were do-it-yourselfers, equipped with bags filled with entertainment options, including our DVD player and a host of movies, Game Boy players and games, quarters for snacks, Batman Band-Aids, and books and magazines to read.

We arrived at our appointment with Dr. Wagner, desperately hoping that he'd tell us that we were clear to go home. In his office, he explained that a recent culture showed some sign of "acid-fast

Gram-positive bacterium." Once again, Allen and I struggled to understand the consequences of words that we had never heard before. Dr. Wagner was hesitant. He said that we could bring Henry home (which was a good thing, since the car was packed and the plane was waiting), but Henry would have to take additional antibiotics. As soon as the appointment ended we headed to the airport, beyond excited to leave Minnesota and close the chapter on our daily struggle between life and death. While we knew that Henry was still vulnerable and would live in isolation from his friends for a full year, we believed the hard part was over.

Thanks to the incredible generosity of the Honeywell Corporation, Henry, Jack, and I flew home on its corporate jet, and were home in a little more than two hours' time. The Honeywell executive on the flight kindly dropped us off in Washington prior to flying to his meeting. This flight was part of the Corporate Angel Network, which arranges free air transportation for cancer and bone-marrow-transplant patients traveling to or from treatments, using empty seats on corporate jets flying on routine business. Flying commercially was out of the question due to poor air quality and too-close proximity to too many people. Henry's eighteen-hour daily IV nutrition, constant diarrhea, and need to avoid people and public places made driving impossible. Allen drove our car home alone.

I thought I would be so grateful and elated to be home. And I was, in a way, as I walked into our house, which was decorated with Welcome Home banners. But I was also surprised to find how out of place I felt; how drained, scared, and lonely I was. I didn't even feel comfortable in my own home. Once a haven, it was now a dirty, scary place that could kill Henry, despite the hours my mom and Abby had spent scrubbing it from top to bottom. The evening of our return, as I waited for Allen to get home, hundreds of friends gathered on our front lawn. The sun had just set and they had all arrived to welcome us back. They were holding glow sticks, bundled in jackets, and serenading us. It was a lovely sight, and a moving and touching gesture. But as I looked out my window, these friends of ours morphed from lifelines into threatening carriers of germs that Henry was too weak to fight. I savored their thoughtfulness and was touched by their kindness, but I wished they'd hurry and leave.

We were too far away from our doctors and the hospital that knew Henry best, and from other people who, through their own life experience, understood ours in a way that everyone we knew from before couldn't. I was overwhelmed. Standing there, behind the curtains, locked inside and away from these people I loved, I realized that I had lost such a big part of who I had been. I doubted that I'd ever get that back. As my brother had always said, I was the life of the family: the spark that started the party; the fun, funny, spontaneous, unworried one. But the failed PGD attempts and the intensity of the fear associated with the transplant had beaten the happy-go-lucky right out of me.

Henry and Jack were excited to see everyone, but I could tell that it was overwhelming even for them. Henry was weak and tired, and while all he wanted to do, I'm sure, was run outside and hug everyone hello, he couldn't. At that point he was taking sixteen doses of medication each day and was on a nutrition pump around the clock. We were up all night and spent our days working hard to help Jack re-enter his world.

I had no time to untangle it all.

Henry's Favorite Things

- Writing his name
- Being naked
- Reading by headlamp
- Making S'mores
- Making (and destroying) forts
- The baseball bat that David Ortiz (Big Papi) signed and gave him
- Visits from the Tooth Fairy

15

SUPER BETTER

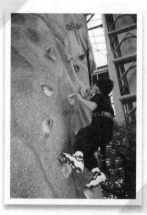

Henry takes it to new heights

$\mathcal{D}$uring the fall of 2000 as Henry continued his bone-marrow-transplant recovery, he and Jack developed an assessment scale of Henry's health status that ranged from "Not Good" to "Super Better." Every day, Henry worked toward Super Better. Thankfully, he was willing to suffer through plenty of Not Good days, recognizing them as a necessary means to an end. He stayed focused on the end game of Super Better, settling for moments or hours of great times here and there, as he worked hard for it to become his way of life.

Two days after we arrived home from Minneapolis, Henry celebrated his fifth birthday. Allen, Jack, Henry, and I wore Batman party hats, ate cake, and broke open a Batman piñata alone in our house—with no one but ourselves to gather all the candy and prizes—as Henry's cousins and friends delivered presents to our front porch and sang "Happy Birthday" in exchange for slices of cake through a barely opened window. Within days, Henry got a fever and was hospitalized at nearby Georgetown Hospital. He got better, and then a few days later he got sick again. So we dumped some stuff into a duffel bag and headed up 95 North, so frazzled that we forgot basics like our driver's licenses and the kids' shoes, and drove to Hackensack, where Henry's longtime hematologist, Dr. Gillio, worked. We never even got a chance to restart the newspaper delivery.

We lived moment to moment, hour to hour, day to day—but never longer than that, in fear of what would happen next. As Henry continued to "recover" from the transplant, we'd spend days, weeks, and months at Georgetown University Hospital in Washington; Johns Hopkins Hospital in Baltimore; Hackensack University Medical Center in New Jersey; and back at the University of Minnesota Children's Hospital, where Henry's doctors tried to unlock the mystery behind his seemingly unending string of complications. His chronic diarrhea; red, peeling skin; low blood counts; and fevers were either a sign of graft versus host disease, infection, or an adverse reaction to one of his many medications. All were a sign of the high-stakes war Henry's body was waging against a recognized foe, Fanconi anemia. Each diagnosis had different, conflicting treatments. A mistaken diagnosis could have fatal consequences. If Henry had graft versus host disease (GVHD), he would require steroids to stifle the donor's cells' attack on his body. But the steroids would make Henry more vulnerable to infection. If he had GVHD and it went untreated, it could escalate from a daily nuisance to a killer. If the cause of Henry's complications was infection and Henry was put on steroids, the infection would worsen and possibly kill him. Until the doctors could find proof that Henry had GVHD, it was too risky to treat him for it. Dozens of skin, gut, and liver biopsies requiring anesthesia, stitches, and hospitalizations failed to offer definitive proof. Because prior to Henry's transplant most children either died by this point or lived better than Henry, our doctors had little experience to draw on.

Chaos reigned as we attempted to straddle our yearning for a normal life (whatever that is) with the reality that the only truly predictable things were fear and loss. In spite of that, we did our very best to savor each day. If anyone had ever told me how hard it would be, or how much pain and suffering my kid would experience, I don't know if I would have had the courage to go through with it. But at this point, there was no turning back. We didn't feel sorry for ourselves or even waste much energy wishing things were different. We just did what we had to do.

In the fall of 2000, I was extremely honored to receive an invitation from Dr. Wagner and his colleague Dr. Jeffrey Kahn, director of the University of Minnesota's Center for Bioethics, to serve as a participant on the University of Minnesota's Working Group on Ethical and Social Issues in Preimplantation Genetic Diagnosis and Hematopoietic Cell Transplantation. In advance of the first meeting, I shared my written account of my experience with PGD with the scientists, ethicists, and legal experts who were charged with debating and proposing guidelines to inform the practice of using PGD to create a child intended to serve as a stem cell donor for another. But transplant-related complications landed Henry in the hospital in Hackensack just prior to the meeting. Allen and I decided that I would stay with Henry and Jack, and Allen would go to Minneapolis as my replacement.

On his way to Minnesota, Allen read my PGD journal for the first time. He knew that I had been documenting our experience, but had yet to read it. As much as he had remained hopeful and optimistic throughout the process, I knew that deep down, of course, he was in tremendous pain. He was in pain because of what he had to watch me put my body through for three years as we tried to get pregnant through PGD. Because he saw the physical and emotional toll every shot, surgery, and disappointment had on me. Because he couldn't be the one to make a physical sacrifice to save Henry. Because he couldn't more easily protect his family and save our son. He was an amazing partner to me and beyond a wonderful father to Henry and Jack, but there was only so much he could take. I noticed how he stopped seeing friends during this time, and how those closest to him often took me aside to ask, "Are you sure he's OK?" I saw how he cringed every time the phone rang, afraid that it would deliver terrible news.

After Allen read my journal during that trip to Minneapolis, he believed that we had an obligation to share our experience as the voice of parents who had responsibly used the technology to try to save a life. Despite our lack of success, we still believed wholly in the promise of PGD. We were certain that the more mainstream PGD became, the more people would misguidedly request its use not only to save lives, but to fill specific cosmetic desires like hair color, eye color, or gender selection. We wanted to speak out, to draw a line in the sand, separate PGD's productive use from the abuse that would threaten to wipe it away. In addition, we both wanted to make the path easier for families who followed behind us, to take away some of the fear and mystery.

Without even mentioning it to me, he sent a copy of my journal to the editor of the *New York Times Magazine.* My journal was the basis of a cover story on July 1, 2001, that Lisa Belkin deftly wrote about Molly Nash and Henry, the promise of PGD, and the consequences of its failure. In the accompanying photos, a healthy Molly was performing ballet, while Henry, in his ubiquitous Batman T-shirt, defiantly bared his transplant-related battle wounds. The *Times* article led to an ABC News *Nightline* feature on February 8, 2002, on our family's journey to the outer limits of science. When these pieces ran, it was clear that Molly was faring far better than Henry and that Henry's fate was still undecided.

When the *Times* piece ran, Henry was still hospitalized at Hackensack. That morning, we bought several copies at the hospital gift shop so each of us could simultaneously read the piece and be prepared for a live chat that day on the *Times*'s website. Allen and I agreed that the piece accurately reflected our experience and represented our family well. One of the reasons we had agreed to be featured in the story was our desire to positively influence the stem-cell debate. We hoped that greater understanding of what was at stake for kids like Henry would encourage the political community to change course and devote significant public resources to support research into potentially lifesaving technologies like PGD. Another reason was to increase knowledge about Fanconi anemia and the importance and availability of prenatal genetic testing and preimplantation genetic diagnosis.

The reaction to the piece was mostly positive. I recall only one chat participant raising the idea that perhaps we should have just let Henry and Molly die. I was one part horrified and the other part shocked that anyone would decline to pursue lifesaving treatment for an innocent child. I don't know if the commenter was influenced by religious beliefs or medical resource allocation concerns or a sense that only the fittest should survive, but I was disgusted, and I pitied the writer and his or her children, if God forbid, there were any.

The producers at *Nightline* were kind enough to share the written reactions to the piece with us. Without exception, the listeners commended us for our courage and supported our efforts to do anything to save Henry. "They should be able to do anything and everything in their power to make Henry well," one commenter wrote. Another kindly inquired if he could donate bone marrow to help Henry. One sent a Valentine's Day card to Henry along with one to Allen and me saying, "I commend you!! Henry is very lucky to have you for his parents. Being a parent myself, I would do anything to save my child." The conservative journalists and think-tank thinkers who had called the Nashes murderers of innocent babies a year earlier were silent.

The overwhelming support paired with the lack of biting criticism put to rest any of my residual concerns about our being branded as reckless parents playing God and indulging in the creation of designer babies. Not only was my worry that protestors would descend upon our home and endanger our lives unfounded, but going public did substantial good. One family wrote to us to thank us for sharing our story as they recognized in Henry's and Molly's faces the facial features of their own child. The mystery of the puzzling set of seemingly unrelated medical issues that afflicted their child was solved through a blood test that revealed Fanconi anemia. Pre-implantation genetic diagnosis provided a pathway out of their despair.

While the world learned of the promise and limitations of PGD, we continued to travel from hospital to hospital, determined to create a positive—and, believe it or not, fun—environment for Henry and Jack. We played balloon ball with blown-up surgical gloves. We watched movies and television. We bought and set up fish tanks in our hotel rooms and filled them with fish with names like One, Two, Red, and Blue. We knew where the best vending machines were in each hospital, where the blanket warmers were, and which showers had the best water pressure. We knew where to take Jack for special outings. And because it so happened that *all* of Henry's hospital rooms were equipped with a Magic Closet, we knew where to get gifts to restock it. Georgetown and Hopkins were near enough to our home that family and friends could easily visit, Jack could go to school, and we could begin to get used to being home. Often, though, only to leave again.

Throughout all of this, Henry still never thought of himself as sick. He was always getting better. If we had time to sit back and take stock of the situation, we may have questioned Henry's reasoning, or even lost our determination to keep fighting. Taken one at a time, each decision we made seemed simple. Henry got a fever, so we would take him to the hospital and put him on antibiotics. Henry couldn't eat, so we inserted a feeding tube. The doctors needed to do yet another surgical procedure to search for a clue to the mystery of Henry's continuing problems, so we allowed them to, hoping we would find an answer with a clear solution and a path to recovery.

We had to do these things to get to Super Better.

*D*uring those years, Allen and I never let go of our dream of having another child. But the fact that we rarely slept in the same room—one of us was at the hospital with Henry, and the other was home or in a hotel or apartment with Jack—made it difficult to do so. That is, until we found ourselves in the midst of a several-months' stay at Hackensack while some of Henry's specialists sought to solve the mystery of his constant diarrhea and unstable platelets. Allen and I figured that our long-term stay in Hackensack had an upside. We could use our frozen embryos that had been in storage for several years at Cornell Hospital to have a baby. I called Dr. Rosenwaks's office and made plans to implant a frozen embryo that

had been tested and diagnosed as Fanconi-free. Each morning for ten days or so, I would take my Lupron injections and travel into New York City at six a.m. for blood tests in preparation for a frozen embryo transfer.

This time around, I wasn't alone.

One year earlier, while we were in New York for my ninth PGD attempt, Allen and I had met, through Dr. Auerbach, Sharon Harari and Yavin Atzmon. They were visiting from Israel with their son Amitai, who, at one and a half years old, had recently been diagnosed with Fanconi anemia. Desperate for information about this rare disease that they knew nothing about, they had come to meet Dr. Auerbach and discuss their options. Many children with Fanconi anemia resemble one another; they have small eyes and are short in stature. When I first met Amitai, I was stunned by how much he resembled Henry. In fact, their whole family immediately felt familiar to Allen and me. Sharon was kind and funny, with fair skin and big curious eyes. Yavin was, like his wife, down to earth and direct. As we sat and talked for a long time about what we had been through—our hopes as well as our disappointments—I felt as if I were looking into the face of the woman I had been three years earlier. Where our eyes had grown tired and fearful, theirs were still energized and hopeful. *Maybe they'll be the ones to benefit from all our hard work,* I thought.

Since that first meeting, Sharon and I had become close. They had returned to Israel, eager to pursue PGD, and we'd spent many hours e-mailing back and forth, having our honest, no-holds-barred "Girl Talks." After our ninth attempt had failed, she was the one I had told right after my family. That's probably because she was the one—the only one, really—with whom I didn't have to explain much, or hide my fears, because she, more than anyone, knew exactly what was at stake. And she was the one to whom, the night of Henry's superhero celebration, I had said what I'd been afraid to

say out loud to anyone else, even Allen: "I am afraid that this might truly be a farewell party."

As I waited to be called into a treatment room for my daily tests, Sharon and I sat together in the waiting room. It was April 2000 and she was in the middle of her third PGD attempt. I passed along a joke I had intended to tell when my PGD was successful. It went . . . "There were three men in the room when I got pregnant. None of them was my husband." I suggested that she could use it when the time came. She laughed.

"There's not a lot of romance to this, is there," she said, and proceeded to tell me the story of giving herself a Lupron shot on the airplane, on her way from Tel Aviv to New York, as someone stood outside the door, knocking loudly. The other women in the waiting room looked curiously at us: two women sitting in a fertility clinic, laughing hysterically.

After I was done with my appointment, I waited for Sharon. I looked around and noted the new upholstery and other updates in the clinic since I had last been there nearly a year earlier. When Sharon joined me, I asked if she liked the décor and new furnishing.

She looked at me curiously and said, "They're nice."

I smiled at her and said, "Thank you. Allen and I paid for the whole thing." It felt good to laugh, rather than the alternative, about all the money we had spent those years.

After the frozen embryo transfer, I took prenatal vitamins and tried to take care of myself, though it wasn't easy to do that while living in the hospital, sleeping (or not) in a chair, eating PowerBars three meals a day, since they exceeded the nutritional content of the entire vending machine, and anxiously waiting for Henry to undergo yet another procedure followed by test results that would inevitably be inconclusive.

A couple of weeks later, the pregnancy test in a bathroom stall at Hackensack was negative. Not long afterward, Allen and I signed

consent forms donating our nearly one hundred remaining embryos to Dr. Hughes for research that would provide answers to other couples, with the hope that no one else would ever have to live through this devastation.

Allen and I determined that the only way to get pregnant was to abandon the use of technology. In the winter of 2001, Henry's ongoing complications led to yet another trip to Minneapolis. Because the stay was likely to be long and Henry wasn't in acute distress, we drove from Washington and got pregnant the old-fashioned way during an overnight stop at a hotel in Cleveland. While in Minneapolis, we learned that we were finally going to have the third child we had spent four years and more than $100,000 trying to produce. My excitement over this longed-for pregnancy and very real fear over Henry's seemingly endless and increasingly serious complications overshadowed my fear that my baby might have Fanconi anemia, but I was worried nonetheless. Allen was certain that the baby would be healthy, that Henry would turn the corner, and that everything would be all right. I wanted to believe him, but to be honest I no longer took comfort in his optimism. I would do my best to remain positive while waiting for confirmation from Dr. Auerbach, who would conduct the prenatal testing ten weeks into my pregnancy.

We were in Minneapolis for one of Henry's post-transplant checkups when Dr. Wagner told us Henry's immune system was finally strong enough for him to go out in public again. It had been seven long, lonely months since the transplant and since he'd been able to do so many of the things he loved. We were determined to do something special to mark the momentous occasion.

We didn't even have to think for a moment about where to go. We chose the most "Henry" destination of all: the Mall of America. Allen, Henry, Jack, and I headed out that day feeling happy and upbeat. Henry's health was improving, spring was approaching, and we just knew we were in for a good day.

After picking up the newest Pokémon and Batman figures at the Warner Bros. store; a visit to the Krispy Kreme factory for some fresh, hot, chocolate frosted doughnuts; and some car racing down the track at LEGO; we headed to Camp Snoopy.

Henry was, at the time, about three-and-a-half feet tall. He wore a protective mask and constantly rubbed his hands with Purell. His central line hung out beneath the bottom of his Batman T-shirt. His face was swollen from the steroids trying to protect his body from rejecting his new bone marrow.

And he was scaling a twenty-five-foot wall.

"You know what, I'm going to do it," he had said, when he first saw the wall at Camp Snoopy.

Before I knew it, Allen and the climbing instructor were staring hard at Henry, scratching their chins, figuring out the best way to negotiate the safety harness around his central line. Then they were knotting the ropes, clipping him in, rubbing his head, and cheering him on. A few seconds later my son was several feet above my head, climbing his way to the top, hand by hand, foot by foot. Everyone cheered, but I was speechless. On his first attempt, he made it up about ten feet. He got about halfway there on his second. With each step, the instructor pulled tightly on the rope and hooted and hollered. It was as if he understood the enormity of what Henry was attempting, despite the fact that they'd known one another for a mere matter of minutes. By his third try, Henry was ecstatic, glee-fully laughing, and ready to call it a day.

"I'll be back," he said to the instructor, unclipping himself from the harness and flashing his famous smile. Then he looked at me. "Not bad, huh?"

"No," I squeaked out, still floored by the courage of my little boy. "Not bad at all."

A few days later, he insisted we go back. He would settle for nothing short of victory. When the instructor saw Henry walking back in, wearing his mask, I thought he was going to cry. With a burst of energy, Henry made it all the way to the top of the climbing wall and rang the buzzer signaling to everyone in Camp Snoopy that he'd summited. Fist in the air, he made his descent. Once on land, he looked me in the eye and said proudly, "I told you I could do it!"

I hugged him tightly. "I didn't doubt it for one second," I said.

*W*hen I was pregnant with Henry, I spent my first trimester shopping for onesies, reading pregnancy books, and decorating his nursery. When I was pregnant with our third child, I spent my first trimester in hospitals in Washington, Baltimore, Hackensack, and Minneapolis, depending on Henry's complication. We probably spent about two hundred days that year in a hospital. I had reduced my work hours to part-time and managed, somehow, to put in the required twenty hours per week, often in the middle of the night while Henry or Jack slept. The demands of my job were primarily strategic planning and writing, both of which were relatively easy to do from the hospital. In many ways, work was a welcome distraction from the places my sleep-deprived mind could wander in the dark of the night, when the only sounds were the continuous pumping of medications into Henry's body and the occasional beep signaling that one medication had run its course and it was time for another.

The Internet start-up company Allen had been working for was one of many victims of the bursting Internet bubble, and its staff reduction included Allen, for whom the demands of the job were hard to fulfill from a distance. Thankfully, my job provided our family with medical benefits and a salary of approximately $40,000 per year, which, when combined with our savings, was enough to live on for the time being. Jack, age four, went to school when we were in DC, but whenever Henry's complications took us out of town, we all stuck together. Often my mom accompanied us when a short stay grew longer, as often happened. While we were on the road, Jack learned the names and classifications of nearly every marine mammal and some basic Spanish, thanks to Dora the Explorer. Henry could recite the lines from nearly every Pokémon episode, and learned to read *Go Dog Go!* Whenever he got to the eponymous page, the four of us pumped our fists three times in the air as we yelled, "Go! Dog! Go!"

Near the end of my first trimester, it was time to find out if the child I carried had Fanconi. My sister, Abby, and I traveled together to a high-risk prenatal testing clinic in Philadelphia recommended by Dr. Hughes for my chorionic villus sampling (CVS) test, which would be sent to Dr. Auerbach for analysis. At the appointment, the genetic counselor explained the risks of the procedure and asked if I wanted to have the updated Jewish genetic screening to see if I was at risk of passing along a deadly disease. She informed me that there were new diseases added to the screening and recommended that I do it. My sister and I looked at each other knowingly. I nodded and signed the consent form.

The day of my test results, I was at my office conducting a performance review for one of my employees when the phone rang. "I have your test results. There is good news and bad news," said the genetic counselor. Before I could ask my employee to leave my office, the counselor gave me the good news. "Your baby boy does not have Fanconi anemia." My forehead in my hands, I took a deep breath, and it felt like the first breath I'd ever taken in my life. "But you tested positive as a carrier of Gaucher disease."

I what?

I was stunned. After all my years doing PGD, how was it possible that I hadn't been tested for everything? I tried to focus on what she was saying—that Gaucher is the most common genetic disease among Ashkenazi Jews, affecting many organ systems like the liver, lungs, and bone marrow—but it was too difficult. I found a pen and a piece of paper. *Gaucher. Like FA, is a recessive gene. If Allen is not a carrier, our children will not inherit it.* I wrote down the address where his blood should be shipped. *Allen. Get tested immediately.* I hung up the phone and asked my employee for some privacy. I put my head down. My tears ran down my cheeks and I watched them form pools on my desk. Allen was at a meeting for a consulting job he had taken to earn money while he searched for full-time work. When I got him on the phone, for the first time that I could remember, Allen broke down and wept right in the middle of a conference room in front of his colleagues. For five minutes, we stayed on the phone, engulfed in silent sorrow.

"I gotta go get tested," he said quietly as he hung up. Within an hour, Allen had had his blood drawn and sent via FedEx to the lab in Philadelphia.

I sat alone in my downtown office and Googled Gaucher and learned, among other things, that its symptoms are evident later in childhood, meaning that Henry and Jack could have it and we wouldn't necessarily know. I tried to focus on the fact that my new baby boy didn't have Fanconi anemia, but it would have been nice if that piece of great news didn't have to compete with the fear that he, Jack, and Henry might have some other horrible disease. I was beyond overwhelmed.

Within days, we learned that Allen was not a carrier of Gaucher, which also meant the kids didn't have it. It was a daunting scare, but, like so many others, I pretty much buried the whole experience in my subconscious.

Despite the relentless wrath of his disease, Henry had the physical and emotional strength to fight back. His ear-to-ear smile and joyous laughter were far more noticeable than his many surgical scars and low platelet-related bruises. After being discharged from

Georgetown, he would ask if we could pick up some lemons and cookie dough on the way home so he could set up his lemonade stand. While I made the cookies, he would create signs featuring new pricing structures that inevitably attracted interest and paying customers. Within days of leaving Georgetown's intensive care unit, he was back on the soccer field with his teammates, dribbling the ball up the field and scoring goals.

The good times were invigorating, strengthening our resolve to keep fighting. But some days were so bad they threatened to crush us.

One of those days was April 25, 2001.

That evening, five-year-old Henry lay on our bed at home in Washington, with Jack, of course. They were watching Nickelodeon as the intravenous antibiotic—Henry's twelfth dose of the day—dripped into his veins. The bed was covered with alcohol wipes, sterile gloves, saline flush, heparin, tortilla chips, an Oreo milkshake, and a bowl of Cheerios. The food sat untouched. Water didn't even taste good to Henry anymore, but Allen and I kept trying everything, hoping to trigger Henry's taste buds to remember something of the pleasure of eating.

I went downstairs and assembled the needles, syringes, and vials of vitamin additives that I needed to mix into Henry's bag of liquid food that would be pumped through the catheter in his chest, into his central venous artery, and through his veins all night long in an attempt to keep him alive. I put what little energy I had into feeling nothing. If I weren't so tired and determined to protect Henry and Jack from the fear that I felt, I would have wept.

A familiar cry distracted me, so I ran upstairs to find Allen carrying Henry to the bathroom for the tenth time that day. Jack, age four, sat on the bed and stuffed an Oreo into his mouth as the Rugrats played on TV. By this time, Allen and I didn't have the will or energy to counter Jack's demands for more cookies and cartoons.

He could eat as many Oreos as he wanted, watch as many cartoons, stay up as long as he wanted. We all indulged ourselves our little obsessions; I collected hand creams and candles; Allen bought CDs. Just a way of staving off reality.

I looked over at Henry. His body was ravaged. It wasn't so much the scars left from his open-heart surgery, or the lung and liver surgeries, or even the catheter that hung limply from his chest. It was the bones; the hip bones and ribs that protruded, naked of fat. He probably looked the same yesterday and for days before, but he had spent most of the past weeks in a bed at Georgetown. I just hadn't noticed; my exhaustion kept me from seeing the obvious.

I took out my camera. I wanted to remember how bad things had become, in case Henry died. I needed to have documentation of the bad times. I thought that after he died, I would remember only the good times, and death in good times didn't make sense. What I recorded on film that night was a child ready to die.

The phone rang. It was Dr. Wagner who, after reviewing Henry's blood work taken at Georgetown earlier that day, confirmed what we suspected. Henry was in grave danger. We had to return to the bone-marrow-transplant clinic in Minneapolis the next day. We had driven before, but we couldn't do it again. It would take too much time, and Henry's IV pump didn't have a car adapter.

I made a list of all the things we had to do to get to Minnesota within twenty-four hours, and Allen and I took them on, one at a time. Allen started by calling and reserving four seats on a flight the next afternoon, which would give us enough time to finish Henry's eight-hour IV nutrition and to give him his first three IV medications, which would take until eleven a.m. It took Allen a while to make the reservation because he had to explain to the airline agent why we didn't have a return date, and why he thought that we should get a good fare, despite the last-minute booking. The airline wouldn't issue our tickets without a return date, so Allen made up a return ·

date and took the agent at her word that all Allen had to do was to submit the $4,800 in receipts to customer service at a later date along with a letter explaining the circumstances to be credited with their best fare. This conversation was followed by similar conversations with car rental and hotel booking agents, each of whom were equally uninterested in the intimate and terrible details of our lives, which Allen had to nevertheless explain in order to receive even a small amount of help.

I pulled out our cooler so we could pack two days' worth of Henry's intravenous medications; then it was on to the suitcases, which were still half-packed from our recent stay at Georgetown. We didn't need to bring clothes for Henry since he had lost a lot of weight and his didn't really fit him anymore; he'd be in hospital pajamas anyhow. I threw in enough clothes for Jack and me to last a week. My belly was growing rapidly—I was approaching my second trimester of pregnancy—so it was impossible for me to predict what size clothing I would need beyond a couple of weeks or so. Allen carefully packed Henry and Jack's favorite movies and computer games for the long days and nights in the hospital.

By midnight, Jack was asleep; Henry was hooked up to his nightly feed; we were packed; and we had reservations for our flight, car rental, and hotel. We had left messages all over town; at Jack's school (he'd be out again), at Georgetown's hematology/oncology clinic (we needed to cancel our appointment the next day), my job (they'd have to do with sporadic e-mails for the next while), and on and on. Our parents were put on notice. They would drive us to the airport, cancel the newspaper, forward our mail, cancel Jack's play dates, clean out our refrigerator.

I couldn't sleep. I was too stirred up with worry and fear, so I paid bills and looked through a stack of pictures from better days. I threw away all the pictures that weren't perfect, just in case Henry didn't return from this trip. Once he died, I didn't imagine that I'd be able to part with anything, even out-of-focus photos. I walked upstairs, past his door, the one with the letters spelling out his name. I wondered whether if he died, we'd ever take the letters down. My mind wandered, horribly, inevitably, to the funeral. I rewrote the eulogy in my head. I'd never be able to deliver it, though, so who would read it? Allen couldn't possibly; maybe my brother. Who would come? Who would officiate? How would I make it through the service, the burial, the day?

The rest of my life?

At some point, I stumbled into bed next to Henry, who was quietly asleep. I woke up some time later, the beeping of his pump signaling the beginning of another day.

By this time, Henry had lost the use of his left side—we had no idea why—and he couldn't walk. Allen carried him through the terminal. If people stared, I didn't notice. Henry finished his IV meds in the airport lounge, so we didn't have to hook him up in-flight. He slept in Allen's lap. Jack and I read about knights and made snakes out of Play-Doh. A few hours later we made it to our hotel, and Allen loaded Henry up in a stroller and Jack pushed him to the clinic. Henry's hematologist, infectious disease doctor, and a neurologist were expecting us.

Three days later, Henry was hooked up to an IV and the four of us were midway through a Pokémon DVD in the hospital's outpatient bone-marrow-transplant clinic. A nurse came into Henry's room and asked the kids if she could take them for a walk. My stomach dropped, and I felt the hot pricks of fear spread from my scalp to my spine. The doctors had never separated us from the kids to deliver news, and there had been plenty of bad news delivered over the years. Henry negotiated with the nurse, extracting a promise to visit the vending machine, and then they were off. Jack pushed Henry in his wheelchair.

Dr. Margie MacMillan appeared. She was part of the transplant team, and one of the experts on FA. She told us, without adornment, that Henry had a mass of unknown origin in his brain. He would be admitted to the hospital immediately and a neurosurgeon would perform brain surgery as soon as possible. I was stunned. Nothing I had ever read, and I had read a lot, ever noted that brain tumors were part of the transplant recovery. I was tempted to run and grab the kids and leave that awful place.

Henry and Jack returned with snacks, and we explained that Henry would have to spend a few nights in the hospital. We told them that Henry would get to take some sleepy medicine, and then the doctors would look inside his head to see why he couldn't walk or play basketball.

He wasn't worried. By this time, he'd had anesthesia so many times, he knew all about it: what flavors he liked best (bubble gum or root beer), what it felt like. It was more important for him to get his left arm back.

Several hours later, a neurosurgeon came to visit me in Henry's fifth-floor hospital room and told me he was able to adjust his schedule so he could perform the brain surgery the following morning. The sooner the doctors knew what was causing the problem, the sooner and more effectively they could treat it.

In the first months of Henry's life, we were able to learn everything about tetralogy of Fallot, the heart problem Henry was born with, and to shop around for the best surgeon at the best hospital to perform his open-heart surgery. When it came to Fanconi anemia, we had years to learn the language and review the research and then to choose the protocol, doctor, and hospital that together would give Henry the best chance of survival. The fact that I knew next to nothing about the brain or neurosurgery or this particular doctor, and wouldn't be able to change that in the fourteen hours between learning of the surgery and handing Henry over to the anesthesiologist, felt incredibly irresponsible, and almost more than I could bear. I didn't even have a computer to Google the doctor, the procedure, the risks, the survival rate. Given that we had no real alternative, our only choice was to follow the advice of Dr. Wagner, in whose hands we had placed Henry's life nearly one year earlier, and to sign the consent forms. At least we had only a limited amount of time to be anxious and scared.

Henry's brain surgery lasted five and a half hours, but it felt more like 19,800 seconds. Allen and I sat in the same waiting room where one year earlier we had learned that Henry had survived the insertion of his first central IV line, signaling the start of his lifesaving transplant. Since then, we had spent hours waiting for confirmation of what was going right, or for clues to solve the mystery of what wasn't. As I sat quietly, I thought, but never uttered out loud, about the risk of stroke, paralysis, and every other awful thing that could happen. I thought about what the doctors might find. I wondered if I would ever be able to talk to Henry again. Brain surgery was hard enough to endure if it alone were the challenge, but on top of a bone-marrow transplant and what felt like an endless stream of biopsies and surgeries, it was more than I could handle. But what choice did we have, really?

"Could you get me a chocolate croissant?" Henry whispered this to me, just seconds after waking from the anesthesia.

"Of course I can," I said as I fought to restrain the tears that threatened to betray my fear and concern as I took note of the enormous bandage that covered Henry's newest battle wound. "I'd love nothing more than to get you a chocolate croissant." I broke the no-cell-phones-in-the-hospital rule and immediately called my mom, who had flown in from Washington to help us. I let her know that the surgery was successful, that Henry was alive, and that he required a chocolate croissant. She and Jack promptly left the Science Museum of Minnesota, where Jack was adding to his deep knowledge of everything dinosaur, and managed to find five chocolate croissants—enough for a celebration.

Five days after Henry's brain surgery, Allen and Jack returned from a trip to LEGO Land in the Mall of America and presented Henry with a LEGO-themed basketball. Henry got that look of determination in his eyes that told you he was about to do something extraordinary. He pushed the button to lower his bed and another to call his doctor. Having assembled everyone, he slowly put his feet on the hospital room floor and steadied himself.

Demonstrating natural showmanship, Henry demanded, "Are you all ready for this?"

In unison, Allen, Jack, my mom, Dr. Wagner, and I all enthusiastically answered his call, "We're ready!"

"Show us what you got, big man," encouraged Allen.

"Get ready for some razzle dazzle! Here it comes!" Henry exclaimed as he proceeded to dribble the basketball with his left hand, which only days earlier he had been unable to lift. Then he did a victory walk around the room, hands in the air, stopping in front of each of us for a much-deserved high-five.

On May 24, 2001, at 4:30 p.m., without a clear diagnosis of what had caused the problem in Henry's brain, or why somehow now it was all right, Dr. Wagner told us we could go home. Scared that he'd change his mind, we rushed to make a ten p.m. flight home to Washington. After five weeks of living out of a suitcase; eating vending-machine and takeout food; removing Jack from his school, friends, and his own life; and handing Henry off to a bunch of strangers who performed brain surgery, a bronchoscopy, an MRI, and three skin biopsies, we couldn't wait to escape.

A few hours later, sitting on the plane, I pulled out my wallet. I still had those two tickets to Funland that I'd stuck in there a year earlier. Funland was just below Disney World on Henry's list of things to do when he got Super Better. For months, through the bone-marrow transplant and the stays in Hackensack and Baltimore, through the return trips to Minnesota, and the brain surgery, every time I took out change for the hospital vending machine or a parking meter, I looked at those increasingly worn green tickets and just hoped like hell that each of my boys would get to use one.

On June 14, less than three weeks after sitting on that plane, we were driving down Route 50 toward Funland with the window down. Because we couldn't fit an IV pole in the car and Henry needed all his daily doses of medication, I extended my arm, gripping Henry's IV bag out the window to ensure that it was positioned properly to flow into his IV line. We arrived at the beach just in time for Funland to open. I disconnected Henry's IV and he was free to go. Once there, I handed Henry and Jack each a ticket and they boarded a boat. There they were: Jack flashing his to-die-for dimples, ringing the bell on his boat like a lunatic; and Henry smiling big, surrounded by the stuffed animals he had won at numerous games in the arcade, unaware of the catheter line hanging out of his shirt and the brain-surgery scar on his head.

We had decided to make a short vacation of this trip, and that night, as we got ready for dinner at Nicola Pizza, home of the famous Nic-o-Boli, Henry turned to me. "Can we go to Funland again tomorrow?" he excitedly asked.

"I can't think of anyplace I would rather be," I said.

We would go to Funland again because at that moment in time, Henry was well enough to go. And because, although we hoped we had seen our last long hospital stay, we knew enough to go when the going was good. Sure, we had to go right when it opened to avoid the crowds, and we had to carry loads of antibacterial wipes, but the next day, we went again and we had a ball. We understood that trips to Funland were part of what Henry was fighting so hard for.

Although most calendars don't officially mark this date, July 6 is, at least in our household, a very important holiday: Henry's Other Birthday. The first time we celebrated this was in 2001, to mark the one-year anniversary of his transplant. In our backyard, among hundreds of water balloons, face paint, and a huge cake, Henry was surrounded by his cousins, aunts and uncles, grandparents, and a few friends. Compliments of the water balloons he had smashed on his own head, Henry's seven-year-old cousin Michael was drenched. He had scribbled with black Magic Marker all over his face and he proceeded to dunk his entire head right into the "Henry Is Great" cake. I thought Henry and Jack were going to pee in their pants. "Remember when Michael smashed his face in the cake?" became the statement that nearly always followed the mere mention of Michael's name. On subsequent holidays, birthdays, and other occasions, Michael's face always found a way into the cake, and Henry and Jack never got tired of it.

As much fun as that day was, nothing could compare to the excitement we felt two months later. When Henry was born, we learned that it was unlikely that he would make it to kindergarten—an event that stood firmly on the other side of open-heart surgery and a bone-marrow transplant that, according to every available piece of information, had very little prospect of success. But on Tuesday, September 4, 2001, the alarm rang at 5:45 a.m. I woke up excited, and went to work starting the first of four IV medicines that Henry, age five, had to take prior to starting his day. At 7:45, Henry put on his backpack and the four of us walked out the front door.

Destination: kindergarten.

As Allen and I watched Henry reunite with Ari and Jake and his other friends from his preschool one year earlier, we snapped some photos and fought back the tears. He had a catheter hanging out of his shirt, was swollen from steroids, and his brain-surgery scar was still visible, but he had made it. Enthralled with all the stuff that makes kindergarten a fantasy world, Henry barely even said good-bye.

Henry's Favorite Things

- Making funny faces at Joe
- Saying "cheese" or *"queso"* right before a photograph
- Getting a hole-in-one in mini-golf
- The color gold, particularly when it is sparkly
- Chasing (and popping) bubbles
- Finding lucky pennies
- Slurpees, preferably a cherry/cola mix

16

BELIEVE

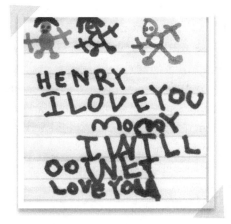

Henry left this on my pillow

$\mathcal{H}$enry was sure about a lot of things. He was absolutely positive that Batman was the best superhero ever, and that Cal Ripken was the greatest living baseball player. He was certain that eating ice cream first wouldn't ruin his dinner, and that what he had with his girlfriend Bella was true love. He was confident that his Tae Kwon Do training would restore his strength and agility. He knew that root-beer-flavored anesthesia, Batman Band-Aids, and the sword that his Papa Sy gave him made all the needle sticks and surgeries hurt a little less.

One thing he wasn't so sure about was the tooth fairy.

"How can she fly all over the world and collect all the teeth?" he asked suspiciously.

"How do you know there is only one?" I replied. "Maybe there are lots and lots of tooth fairies," I posited.

"Good point," he said.

During his first few months in kindergarten, Henry's friends started to lose their teeth. But not Henry. Henry's teacher took advantage of the growing number of missing teeth to reinforce her lesson in the use of tally marks. Every week an increasing number of gap-toothed smiles produced more tally marks, but not one of them was for Henry. His teeth wouldn't budge. He tried wiggling them. He tried wishing them loose.

"Try now," he said, asking me to feel how loose his tooth was.

"It's a little looser than yesterday," I replied. "Definitely." But in truth, there was nothing doing.

To make sure he was prepared for the big day whenever it came, I bought Henry a small, light blue, silk tooth fairy pillow. It smelled of lavender. The pillow had a little pocket sewn on with small white sequins, and featured the black outline of a tooth. When Henry's first tooth fell out, he planned to put it in the pocket and then put the small pillow under his big pillow in the hopes that the tooth fairy would pay up just like she did for all his friends.

"Come on, you can tell me. Is she real?" he asked at the dinner table one evening, still a little unconvinced.

"She visited me when I was a kid, how about you, Allen?" I replied.

"You bet," he said.

"How much did she give you?" Henry asked. Clearly the kids at school were talking.

"I hear the going rate is five dollars for the first tooth," I said.

"Wow," he responded.

Henry's smile in his kindergarten graduation photo showed a mouth full of baby teeth.

By that summer, Henry's doctors had determined that they needed to extract five of his teeth. The radiation and chemotherapy he had undergone to prepare for the transplant had predictably begun to cause tooth decay. Henry's still-compromised immune system was too weak to fight infection, making it critical to remove the teeth immediately.

"Will it still count?" Henry asked on the way to have surgery at Georgetown where, in addition to removing five teeth, doctors would also insert a tube to stem his ongoing weight loss, yet another harrowing and enduring transplant complication.

"Of course," I said.

"How will she know where to find me?" He sounded pretty worried.

"Trust me," I said. "She will. She's magic."

An hour or so later, Henry's doctors found Allen and me in the hospital waiting room. The surgeries were successful they told us, before presenting us with Henry's teeth.

"We got the teeth, big man," said Allen as Henry awoke from his anesthesia. We all went upstairs to settle into Henry's fifth-floor hospital room for yet another multiday stay. As night approached, Henry stuffed the teeth into the pocket of his tooth fairy pillow, which he carefully tucked under his hospital-issued pillow. Eventually he fell asleep.

As they did whenever he was in the hospital nearby, Henry's grandparents came to visit. Pop Pop Teddy was first. Figuring that Henry deserved some extra cash, given the anesthesia and all, he rolled up $10 per tooth—or $50—and tucked it into the pocket. Nana and Papa Sy offered up a matching gift and tucked in another

$50. When Henry woke up that morning, he reached under his pillow, grabbed the $100, and exclaimed, "She found me!"

The next day Henry shared his news with Jack. "Jackie, the tooth fairy gave me a hundred dollars!" Jack started wiggling his teeth that afternoon, hoping the tooth fairy would find him soon. With a going rate of $20 per tooth, he figured it was a better way to make money than a lemonade stand.

Within days, Henry was discharged from the hospital. Before heading home, Henry insisted that we go to Best Buy, where he procured two new Nintendo Game Boy Advance players, one for him and one for Jack, compliments of his tooth fairy bonanza.

Back home, he couldn't wait to get back to school. By late fall of 2001, it was his favorite place. He was so excited when it was his turn to be Door Holder, one of the special jobs his teacher doled out. He thought being Milk Helper was pretty great too. And when the time finally came to have his central line removed, he brought it to school in a plastic bag to share at Circle Time.

"This is my line," he explained to his gaped-mouth classmates. "I finally got it out." Then he passed it around the circle. The kids were a bit baffled by the piece of white plastic tubing Henry dangled in front of them. Apparently they hadn't noticed it hanging out from under his T-shirt for the past year. Later, when I asked his teacher, Mrs. Singer, how the children had responded, she explained that the kids—and everyone else at the school for that matter—didn't look at Henry as being sick, just as a really nice friend, and a really determined student. When Henry would get tired, he would go to the school office and lie down with a blanket and pillow in the spot his teacher had created for him to take a nap. When he was done, he would get up, smile, and say to the school receptionist, "Gotta go to class. See you later!"

And then off he would run.

The only job he was never assigned in school was that of the Get

Well Card Helper. This special job was reserved for the times when Henry had to be absent for days and weeks at a time. One student would be asked to collect all the handwritten cards and pictures drawn by the others, put them in an envelope, and get them ready to send to Henry. This job was a quality-of-life saver for Henry, and was, unfortunately, needed a lot more than any of us would have liked.

Henry's Favorite Things

- Climbing trees
  - His bright blue Pokémon bicycle
    - Mastering his white-belt basics
  - Patagonia long underwear
- Lightsabers
  - Wearing flip-flops
- Joe

17

A Moment in Time

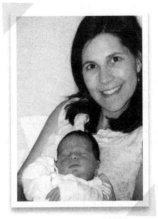

Joe, joy and calm amidst the storm

𝓜osquitoes love Jack.

Therefore, it didn't worry me too much when Jack started to scratch his belly and the first couple of bites popped up. "I'm itchy" just didn't rank high on the list of concerns in our house, or probably anyone else's for that matter, especially one week after September 11, 2001, when it felt like the whole world was falling apart.

An hour later, Jack was still scratching, so I lifted up his shirt and noticed that he had about a dozen red bumps on his belly. I gave him some Benadryl and put some calamine lotion on the bites and he rejoined Henry, who was watching Pokémon 2000 for the two-thousandth time. I returned to the kitchen where Allen and I resumed our position in front of our small black-and-white TV, watching the jaws of death make its way carefully through the pit of destruction that was once the World Trade Center. The camera focused on the sad, shocked faces of family members walking through the streets, cradling pictures of missing loved ones whose lives they didn't even have a chance to save. Watching this horror, for a few moments I forgot about my problems.

But then something struck me: it didn't seem right. "Why are the bites only on Jack's stomach?" I asked Allen. Before he could answer, I added, "I don't have any, and I always get more than anyone." Jack and I were in the backyard blowing bubbles together the night before. Allen said he'd go take a look.

While Allen was in the other room, my mind started to wander. Could it be a rash? But Jack had never had a rash on his body before. We hadn't used any new detergent and he hadn't eaten any new foods.

Could it be a bad thing—*the* bad thing? Could it be chicken pox?

"No!" I yelled to Allen in the other room, as if we had been having a conversation about the possibility. "No way. There is no way that is chicken pox!"

Jack had gotten vaccinated against chicken pox four years earlier when he turned one, mostly to spare him from getting the virus, but also to protect Henry. When the chicken pox vaccination, Varivax, first became available in 1995, it was an enormous blessing for parents of immune-compromised children like Henry, because a disease like chicken pox can cause bacterial infections, such as pneumonia, which his body was too weak to fight. We vaccinated

Henry and Jack at our first opportunity, and every teacher and friend knew to call us immediately if they heard of a case of chicken pox, so we could watch and pray that it passed over our house.

"I think it's just a bunch of bug bites," Allen said, walking back into the kitchen. I wasn't so sure. I turned off the television and went straight to my computer. While I searched the Internet to confirm that Jack could not possibly have the chicken pox, Allen called our pediatrician to describe Jack's symptoms: itchy red bumps that resemble bug bites, no oozing, no bleeding, and no fever. Jack was a little uncomfortable and tired, but otherwise was fine. They couldn't make a diagnosis over the phone, so Allen drove Jack to the doctor for an assessment while I called Dr. Gillio to see what we needed to do if Jack had the chicken pox.

As I waited for Dr. Gillio to come to the phone, I continued to Google "chicken pox" and frantically looked for more information: What chicken pox looked like. Whether you could get it after being vaccinated or from someone who had been vaccinated. Whether Henry's bone-marrow transplant could have rendered his vaccinations useless. How chicken pox were transmitted. How they were treated. Whether there was anything we could do at this point other than wait. And if getting them really meant Henry could die.

As I was reading and printing and panicking and waiting to hear from Allen and Jack, Dr. Gillio got on the phone. I described Jack's symptoms. Since Dr. Gillio was more than two hundred miles away in Hackensack, he couldn't make a diagnosis. He did, however, tell me about the availability of a vaccination called VZIG (varicella-zoster immune globulin) that held the promise of protecting Henry from getting the chicken pox if in fact Jack had it. Henry would have to get vaccinated within ninety-six hours of exposure, before any symptoms appeared. After he got the VZIG, we would have to wait ten to twenty-one days to see if it worked. During that time, Henry could take IV acyclovir, an antiviral medication he had taken for a year post-transplant, which should strengthen his ability to fight the disease. To top it off, in the event a vaccination and yet another IV drug weren't enough, Henry would need to avoid Jack for a week or so, just to be completely safe.

If Jack had the chicken pox, then he had been contagious one or two days before the rash appeared, which included the day before, when they made forts in their bunk bed and played for hours in each other's sheets and blankets. The reality is that we didn't know if Jack had the chicken pox, and wouldn't know for certain before the ninety-six-hour window was shut. On the phone, Allen and I weighed the risk of getting the vaccine if Jack didn't have the chicken pox (yet another shot) versus not getting the vaccines if he did (possible death).

I could barely speak. "After surviving heart surgery, brain surgery, and a bone-marrow transplant, he couldn't possibly die of chicken pox, could he?" I finally managed.

We hung up and I called Dr. Aziza Shad, Henry's doctor at Georgetown's hematology/oncology clinic, to see if they had a supply of VZIG, which they did. I asked them to prepare the dosage and to call Corum, our home health-care delivery service, and ask them to send us a supply of IV acyclovir. I called Allen again, who had just sat down with Jack in the sick-kid waiting room at the pediatrician's office. They hadn't seen Jack's doctor yet, but Allen agreed with me that we'd better get Henry to Georgetown so if the pediatrician had any question at all about the possibility that Jack had the disease, we could get Henry vaccinated right away.

"It looks like you're going to have to get a shot today to make sure you don't get the chicken pox," I said to Henry, while we played chess.

"Oh, man," he said. "That's no fun."

"Well, let's get it done now, so we can get to the toy store before it closes. I think this calls for a special treat, don't you think?"

He was so used to getting stuck with needles by that time that he was generally OK with it, particularly if it would lead to the acquisition of a new toy. We got in the car and drove to Georgetown so we'd be there before the hematology/oncology clinic closed for the day. While we were on our way, Allen called to say that the pediatrician suspected that Jack had a mild form of chicken pox, the kind you get if you fall outside the 70 to 90 percent likelihood that, once vaccinated, you won't get it at all.

"Jack's being sent to a pediatric dermatologist in the same building to get a second opinion," Allen told me.

Just as I hung up, a horrifying thought crept into my head. I was more than eight months pregnant. Though I had somehow failed to absorb the information at the time, I remembered that when I was searching the Internet an hour earlier for any information about the most serious risks associated with chicken pox, I saw something about pregnant mothers and babies and birth defects and death. I called Allen back and asked him to go back and ask the pediatrician what we needed to do to protect our baby and me.

My mind was flooded with another set of questions: Did I have to avoid Jack and Henry? Did I need to get the same vaccination as Henry? Was it safe to get it so far along in my pregnancy? Did we need to give the baby the vaccination as soon as he was born? Was I protected since I'd had the chicken pox as a kid? Was the baby protected for the same reason? Was Jack going to be OK? Was Henry going to die? Were things ever going to get easier? Could I take even one more day of this shit?

But Henry was sitting in his car seat right behind me, so I didn't ask any of them. Instead, Henry and I talked about which superhero was cooler—Batman or Batman Beyond. I preferred the old-school style, but Henry made a good case for Batman Beyond.

"Mom, his Batsuit is so cool. He can shoot batarangs and he can fly. Come on!"

For the first time in my life, I was afraid of Jack. Henry and I arrived at the clinic at Georgetown's Lombardi Cancer Center just before closing time, where we learned that the VZIG was actually two shots, not one. I called Allen for an update on Jack. Allen was in with the dermatologist, who was fairly sure that Jack had the chicken pox, but could not say definitely without a blood test and skin biopsy, which involved needles and stitches—the equivalent of torture to Jack.

Thankfully, the results wouldn't be available in time to help us decide whether to treat Henry, so we could spare Jack. If we had more time, we would have had to balance the pain and discomfort to Jack with the consequences of not doing it at all. The treatment for Jack if he did or did not have the chicken pox was essentially the same—oatmeal baths, Benadryl, calamine lotion, or none of the above, depending on how bad he felt. So, it wouldn't feel so great subjecting him to a blood test and skin biopsy, which we knew from experience with Henry involved using something that looks like a small apple corer to extract a chunk of skin, leaving a hole that required stitches. No matter how many times Jack had sat and watched Henry get poked and stitched up, he had never warmed to the idea of having to be the patient himself.

"Let's just get it over with," Henry said. He had quickly decided that it would be best to get both shots at the same time and just get it over with, so we could get to the toy store before it closed. "Two shots, two presents," he said. "And one for Jack, too," he added.

So Henry's two nurse friends, Suzanne and Kathy, each armed with a shot, stood next to me and Henry and we all did the countdown: "Five, four, three, two, one. Go!" On the way out, Suzanne asked Henry if he'd go on another date with her to Cactus Cantina. "How about tomorrow?" he answered.

And so the decision was made. We would have to wait through the twenty-one-day incubation period to see if it worked. In the meantime, Henry had scored a date out of the deal.

Dr. Shad explained that I wasn't at risk since I'd already had the chicken pox, and neither was the baby as long as he remained in my body. Allen got similar information from the pediatrician and Jack's new dermatologist. I wasn't due for a few weeks, so we still had time to get more information about the risk to the baby once he was born.

As promised, Henry and I headed to Tree Top Toys, a local toy store, to get two treats each for Henry and Jack. Henry picked the card game Skip Bo and a spin-art kit. He thought Jack would like a new several-hundred-piece Knight's Kingdom LEGO set. Henry and I returned to an empty house. I packed a bag for Allen and Jack, and left it along with the LEGOs and a love note on the front porch. Allen and Jack picked up the goods and relocated to my parents' apartment. They planned to stay there for the next five days while Jack was contagious and, thus, the most significant threat to Henry's life. At some point during the waiting period, I would have a baby, and we and our family and friends would find a way to make it through the chaos that continued to define our life.

After Henry fell asleep, I sat alone in the dark in our kitchen and turned on the television, only to learn that in addition to the horrifying terrorist acts that had occurred in New York and Washington and those that may yet occur, potentially lethal letters containing anthrax spores were circulating throughout the country with the potential to deliver death right through our mail slot. Within days, neighbors throughout Washington were sealing their mailboxes, preferring to collect their mail in plastic bins outside their homes, which they would go through wearing plastic gloves.

I didn't know what to be scared of anymore.

I stayed home from my job, took my prenatal vitamins, did spin art, and played hundreds of games of Skip Bo, Uno, and Blink with Henry. Each afternoon I looked through the mail spilling into our foyer, convinced that no one would be that heartless.

Three days later, Allen and I couldn't take the separation any longer. Jack's chicken pox—or bug bites or rash (we never did find out definitively what he had)—never got any worse than they were the first day we noticed them. In fact, they were smaller. The itching was gone and the blisters never came. So Allen and Jack moved into our basement, where they ate their meals, watched movies, slept in sleeping bags, and tried to make a good time of it for another few days. Henry and I lived upstairs, and we all spent a lot of time shouting up and down the basement stairs. After the kids fell asleep, Allen and I met in the kitchen in front of the television. We watched the firefighters search for bodies, bereaved family and friends walk the streets of New York with fliers featuring pictures of lost loved ones, and reports of yet another anthrax-laden letter. We held hands across the table, but we didn't speak. We were too worn out and overwhelmed to say much of anything.

I awoke to an e-mail from Sharon in Israel. She was writing to share with us, Mark Hughes, Arleen Auerbach, and Zev Rosenwaks the most wonderful news: Their third PGD attempt had worked. She was pregnant.

Three long years of struggle, living under the shadow of death have finally reached a dramatic turning point for our family. We will wake up tomorrow morning with renewed hope. This is a celebration of scientific ingenuity, state of the art medicine, and the most profound expression of human collaboration. Through this long journey yet to be continued, Yavin and I were always guided by a combination of ideas:

A focused attitude of doing everything possible regardless of geographic, financial, physical and emotional difficulties, and a deep understanding of the word "hope" and its role in our life. We always felt that although the outcome of this effort would be crucial, the road we took and the decisions we made along the way would help us get through life in one piece even if we fail. This sober point of view makes us especially happy and relieved today, knowing that thanks to all of your work and effort our future seems to be so much brighter.

Our warmest thoughts are with our very special friends— Laurie and Allen—who not only paved the way in a very practical manner, but also reminded us again and again what real optimism and determination are all about. The Nashes, whom we have never met nor spoke to, helped us believe this can really work when we were confronting obstacles along the way.

We send our deepest thanks and appreciation halfway around the globe for all that you have done for our family, and a special thanks in advance on behalf of all those families that will be fortunate enough to be as lucky as we were.

I cried when I finished reading the e-mail. It was exactly what I would have written, I thought, were I the one with this news to share.

The next day, Sharon left me another message. "I can't stop thinking about you," she said on my voice mail. "This never would have happened to us were it not for you and Allen. It's as simple as that. You are the mother that I want to be to my kids. You do every-thing. You provide laughter and safety, fight so hard, and give so much love. I hope you are well, and that Henry is getting better."

*H*enry was not getting better.

After the contagious period was over, our life returned to the state it was in prior to September 18, when the fear of the pox started. Two weeks later, our respite was interrupted by a fever and infection that sent Henry to the hospital. He had a recurrence of MRSA (methicillin-resistent Staphylococcus arueus, or staph infec-tion) at the site of his central venous catheter, through which he continued to receive intravenous medication, fluids, and blood trans-fusions. This infection develops in hospital patients with weak im-mune systems who have tubes going into their bodies. In other words, in people like Henry. The infection required the doctors to surgically remove the line and replace it with an IV, through which he could receive antibiotics, along with the acyclovir that he was still taking to protect him from the chicken pox.

Midway into Henry's one-week stay at Georgetown, nature took its course and I gave birth to our third son, Joe Strongin Goldberg, at Sibley Memorial Hospital, less than five miles away. Amidst the complexity of our life and in the world, Joe came to us easily. We tried to produce him through a mix of scientific breakthrough and miracle, but instead he showed us that sometimes the best things in life come simply and naturally. So we chose a simple yet strong name for our baby boy.

Joe was born during a scheduled Cesarean section and entered the world in perfect health early on the morning of October 6, 2001. At the time of Joe's birth, my mom was with Henry at Georgetown, Jack was at my sister's house nearby, and Allen was at my side to wit-ness the birth of the baby we had wanted for five long years. Henry met his baby brother Joe through a video made by Allen, the same way I met Henry six years earlier. Jack and Allen spent their days shuttling back and forth from Henry's hospital room to mine. I lay in my hospital bed recovering from my C-section, holding tight to Joe, desperate to protect him from terrorists, anthrax, chicken pox, staph infections, and all the other crap in the world.

Henry's Favorite Things

- Watching Looney Tunes cartoons
- Chasing Snow White around Disney World
- Going to birthday parties
- Whistling with acorns
- Eating Rolos
- His number 23 Michael Jordan jersey
- Pumpkin patches

18

FATE

Henry, the real boy who lived

enry was two when he put on his first Batman costume. From that day on, or at least until the time we left for Minneapolis for his transplant, he barely took it off. By that point, he didn't need it anymore. He had achieved superhero status in his own right. Like Batman, Henry's special powers were his strength and intelligence, which he developed through hard work and training. While Batman faced numerous adversaries, including the Joker, Ra's al Ghul,

Riddler, Two-Face, and Poison Ivy, Henry faced only one, Fanconi anemia. Henry was a master of illusion. He made everyone—perhaps me most of all—believe that anything was possible. The only thing that seemed impossible was that inside his beautiful body, every single cell possessed a genetic defect so deadly that one day he would die. Despite all our hope, love, and persistence; Henry's courage; and the best the medical profession had to offer, the impossible happened. Seven years, one month, two weeks and two days after he was born, Fanconi anemia took my son away. A short trip to Minnesota for a tune-up turned into a long farewell.

But it started back home.

It was August 2002. Jack and I were playing Monopoly in the basement one warm and quiet morning. I landed on Boardwalk and was trying to decide whether to buy it, thereby sealing my victory, or passing on it and going easy on him. All things considered—he was five years old and his older brother, Henry, was so sick—I figured he could use a break. So I passed up my opportunity to make a fortune in real estate, and it was his turn. As Jack rolled the dice, I told him I was just going to run to check on Henry, who was napping in my bed. Ten-month-old Joe was peacefully napping in his crib.

Upstairs, I leaned over to give Henry a kiss on his cheek. He didn't even flinch. I pulled down the covers. His emaciated body was deep purple, his eyes had rolled back in his head, and he did not appear to be breathing. I screamed at him to get up, to breathe, to talk. Nothing. I shook him. Nothing. I screamed downstairs to Jack, urging him to hurry, to come help me. Then I remembered that he was only five, and I hoped he hadn't heard me. I fell onto the bedroom floor. I startled myself and crawled across the floor to the phone and dialed 911, screaming at Henry to wake up, and at the operator that my son had died or was dying. I didn't know where my husband was, I was all alone, and that he couldn't die now.

"Please help me," I sobbed into the phone. "Don't let him die. Not now. Not after everything we have been through!"

I hung up, and tried to regain my senses. Allen. He was on his way to the airport to pick up his father, who was returning home from a trip to Alaska that he had taken with Allen's sister Jennifer and her family. It was the first time he had left town since, to all of our great sadness, Allen's mother, Phyllis, had died a few months earlier. We were all reeling from the pain of her death, which occurred in the middle of one of Henry's hospitalizations for yet another transplant complication. With three children, one a newborn, another a healthy five-year-old, and a very ill six-year-old, we had no time to cry. Until now. I wept into Allen's voice mail and pleaded with him to come home. I got up off the floor and stroked Henry's hair and begged him to wake up. Then I remembered Jack and Joe. I needed to find someone to take care of them so I could get in the ambulance with Henry. I couldn't leave them home alone. I couldn't send Henry off in an ambulance alone. I called my neighbor, Cati Bannier, who took advantage of a pause while I gasped for breath to ask if I had put a mirror by Henry's mouth to see if he was breathing. For a moment I stopped to wonder how she even knew an esoteric thing like that. The next thing I knew, her husband, Chuck Lane, was downstairs letting the police in.

Henry's pulse barely registered. We did not have enough time to wait for an ambulance to arrive, so I wrapped Henry's limp, naked body in my bedspread and tried to pick him up, but I couldn't. A policeman carried him downstairs, put him in the squad car, and we raced to Georgetown, only a few blocks away, siren blaring. We rushed through the emergency room doors—where we had been many times before—and the waiting team of doctors, nurses, and techs grabbed Henry, threw him on the operating room table, stuck a breathing tube down his throat, and inserted IVs that pumped medication into both arms. I collapsed on the floor in the corner of the room.

I didn't know if Henry was dead or alive.

I watched as a chest X-ray was taken and tossed up on the wall. The tech stared in disbelief and exclaimed, "What has this kid had done to him?" From my position on the emergency room floor, I stopped sobbing long enough to rattle it all off, slightly above a whisper.

Tetralogy of Fallot open heart surgery thumb removed bone marrow transplant a lung biopsy two liver biopsies brain surgery two Hickman catheters a G-tube.

Please, I added. *Don't let my boy die.*

I sat on the floor, waiting for Allen. We had spoken at some point, although I could barely recall when. I told him that I didn't know whether Henry was alive. I told him to come, as soon as he could. After we had talked, a nurse had called Allen, urging him to get quickly to the hospital. He would be needed to help me make "difficult decisions." Allen heard this as good news. At least Henry was still alive. Allen voiced concern that he might be stopped by the police since he was driving 90 mph in a 45 mph zone and passing cars on the left and on the right. The nurse said that wouldn't be a bad thing—the police would get him to the hospital even faster.

Allen arrived. Henry was unconscious, on a ventilator, his life still in jeopardy. Hours later, Henry was transferred to a room in the pediatric intensive care unit where he lay lifeless but for the ventilator pumping oxygen into his lungs.

Allen came close to me, and I saw the anguish in his eyes.

"I have to tell you something," he whispered, his voice cracking into pieces. He told me, confided in me, that although he was sure that he had given Henry the right dose of morphine before heading out to pick up his father—he was as diligent a nurse to Henry as I was—he was now unsure of himself and possibly, even probably, he thought this was all his fault. He was to blame. My reassurances fell on deaf ears. I couldn't talk him out of that fear then, or today.

The next day Henry woke up surprised to find himself in the hospital surrounded by doctors, nurses, and connected to a bunch of machines. He took in the scene.

"What happened?" he asked.

The sound of his voice and the alertness in his eyes told me all I needed to know—that his brain was in as good working order as ever. I told him the exciting tale of how his heart had stopped briefly and how we got to ride in a police car with the siren blaring, and how his superpowers had been activated and he started breathing again. I balanced my desire to tell the truth while disguising the death-defying nature of the incident. I didn't want him to be scared to take a nap again for fear he would never wake up.

Henry listened intently and said with a smile, "I'm like Harry Potter. I'm the boy who lived."

I don't know if it was my maternal instinct, the doctors' skills, Henry's resolve, or just plain luck, but Henry did not die that day.

In fact, he started to feel better. A few days after surviving this experience, Henry's physician, Dr. Shad, stopped by his room on a Friday evening, on her way out for the night.

"Have a good weekend, Henry," she said with a smile.

"That's easy for you to say," he responded. "How can I have a good weekend when I'll be here in the hospital the whole time?"

After a brief pause, he added, "I have an idea. You know what will make it better? My friend's having a birthday party. Maybe I could break out of here for a while and head over there."

Dr. Shad, one of Henry's most compassionate doctors, looked carefully at him and then at me. "That does sound fun," she said. "Do you think you can keep your mask on the whole time?"

Henry's smile grew larger as he furiously nodded his head.

"And do you promise to wash your hands really, really well?"

Two days later, Henry was at his friend Rachel's sixth birthday party. With all of his friends from school, he ate cake, helped open the gifts, and ran as fast as he could—which was a lot slower than all the other kids—through an obstacle course created for the occasion. When he finished, everyone high-fived him. He left with his goodie bag and filled with renewed determination to spend less time in the hospital and more time at parties.

Two weeks later, Allen and I drove him and Jack to school for their first day in first grade and kindergarten respectively. Henry showed Jack around the kindergarten classroom, introducing him to the teachers and classroom turtle, Speedy, and then hurried off to see all his friends.

Henry started first grade with much enthusiasm. "At school I like to go to PE," he wrote in the journal he kept in class. A later entry had a picture of a pumpkin that Henry had taken with his new Polaroid camera. He signed it "Harry." Like millions around the world, Henry loved Harry Potter and felt a special connection to another boy who had survived against all odds.

Henry's note under the photo read: THE BOY WHO LIVED TOOK THIS PICTURE.

Within days, Henry was hospitalized with yet another transplant-related complication. We had all along sent Henry and Jack to a small private school where everyone knew one another and the school made it a priority to protect Henry. The parents of kids in his class had agreed to call us if they observed any signs of illness in their children so we could keep Henry home from school. Obviously, there was a risk that a child could have the flu or chicken pox before the parent realized, but we were determined to weigh that risk against the clear benefit to Henry of going to school and being with friends.

Not long after this hospitalization, Drs. Shad and Wagner agreed that Henry's health had deteriorated to a point where he could no longer attend school. His immune system was not strong enough to fight off the common germs that are a natural part of the school environment. Henry spent the month of October in isolation at home, with the exception of sneaking out to see Bella the evening of his seventh birthday.

Something just didn't seem right to me. It had been more than two years since Henry's transplant, and he still needed blood transfusions. That fall, his inability to grow and thrive had required a feeding tube into which I administered all his nutritional needs. But despite the fact that he was "eating" plenty, he was shrinking in size. In 2002, Henry had gone from wearing size 7 in the spring to 6 in the summer, and 5 and then 4 by his seventh birthday in October. While Henry was still bigger than our baby Joe, Jack towered over him. Throughout the year, rarely had more than a week gone by without an infection and hospitalization. We never even bothered to unpack our bags, as we had come to expect late-night fevers and dashes to emergency rooms. Our optimism kept us going to the beach or on vacation when we could, so we got to know the emergency room staff at hospitals in New York City; Lewes, Delaware; and Fort Myers, Florida. I had long since given up going to the office, settling for working online for my required twenty hours per week to keep our health insurance, which protected us from financial ruin. Allen didn't bother to look for a full-time job anymore, since he couldn't even count on being able to show up for an interview. Henry's medical-bill folder went from filling up a desk drawer to occupying three large storage tubs.

But none of that led me to conclude that it was time, yet again, to return to Minnesota. Instead, it was my conversation with Henry early one morning in November 2002, when he asked if we could talk about the good old days when he was three. He wanted to talk about his dates with Bella especially, like the time he went to her ballet recital with her family and brought her a bouquet of flowers. The only other time I remember having a conversation like that was with my ailing grandmother just before she died. We laughed as we remembered the good times in an effort to stave off the reality that her life would end at any moment. That was the last time I saw her.

Allen and Henry went to Minnesota first. We decided that I would remain home with Jack and Joe, so Jack could go to school and Joe, who was still a baby, could avoid the harsh Minnesota winter weather and hospital-borne germs that could pose a threat to his young immune system. Dr. Wagner would examine Henry and let us know whether my instincts were on to something or if, as everyone else believed, this was just another bump in Henry's rocky road to recovery. Dr. Wagner wanted them to stay a few days.

Allen viewed this as a boys' getaway, so upon arriving in Minneapolis he started planning the fun. He bought two tickets to a college football game between the University of Minnesota and my alma mater, the University of Michigan. Over the years, I had gotten everyone hooked. Henry and Jack were proficient at yelling "Go Blue!" from an early age. Within days of their arrival, Henry got a fever and was hospitalized, and Jack and I flew to Minnesota. One week later, my mom and Joe joined us, and we all moved into the local Ronald McDonald House. Needless to say, Allen and Henry never got to see the inside of the Metrodome on that trip.

The Get Well Card Helper in both Henry's and Jack's classes

got to work, and while we were in Minneapolis that fall, Henry and Jack received many packages from school filled with pictures, cards, and notes from friends and teachers. "Henry. I love you. I miss you very, very much. Please come back to school soon," said Emily. This sentiment was echoed by kids in nearly every grade of Henry and Jack's small Jewish day school in Washington.

Allen and I switched off nights at the hospital while the other slept in our one-bedroom apartment with my mother, Jack, and Joe. One week led to another, so we enrolled Jack in the Minneapolis Jewish Day School, where he would join friends he had made when we first arrived in Minneapolis years earlier. With temperatures well below freezing, my friend Susie shipped a box filled with hats, gloves, snow pants, and winter boots for all of us. Allen's family flew to Minneapolis to join us for Thanksgiving dinner at Ronald Mc-Donald House, which was warm and generous and sad and lonely.

Allen brought some new music and with it, new cheer into Henry's room, compliments of Dan Zanes's *Night Time!* With songs like "Smile Smile Smile," about how just thinking of a special someone makes you smile; and "Firefly," about how those little bugs bring the magic of summer to the air; and "Side by Side," about how none of the bad things matter much whenever we're together, it was as if Dan Zanes wrote the whole album with Henry in mind. Dan Zanes calls it "nighttime music, firefly music, shadow music, rainstorm music, bat music, streetlight music, dinner music, moon and stars music, flashlight music, or dream music." I call it "Henry music"—and whenever I hear it, I cry.

I knew Henry was nearing the end on December 6, 2002, when Allen and I negotiated a one-hour leave from the hospital in a desperate attempt to remind him of some of the pleasures of life. Allen, Henry, Jack, and I took a quick trip to Toys "R" Us, carefully placed

Henry's shrunken body into a shopping cart, and bought him the new robotic Star Wars R2D2 he had been longing for.

He didn't even crack a smile. Instead he begged to return to the hospital for more morphine to diminish the excruciating pain.

That night as the Hanukah candles in his hospital room extinguished, Henry began to gasp for breath. Around midnight, he sat in my lap and I enveloped him in my arms as we made our way in a wheelchair through the deserted, lonely hospital corridors to the radiology department. In the middle of the night, I called Allen, who was with Jack, Joe, and my mom at the Ronald McDonald House nearby, to let him know that things were deteriorating and I was scared. In a matter of hours, Henry lost the capacity to enjoy even a good moment, then the ability to breathe on his own, then he lost consciousness.

The last words Henry said to me were "Mom, this is a very bad last night of Hanukah."

I made my final desperate call to Allen, who stood gloveless outside the Ronald McDonald House chipping away at the ice on the windshield of our rented minivan in the subzero Minneapolis cold, asking him to come immediately. Allen arrived as I was screaming down the hall for someone to help me as the code red alarm blared from Henry's room. Over the next several days, Allen's father and my father, our siblings, Allen's friend Bill, and my aunt flew to Minneapolis to visit and help us survive yet another quiet, horror-filled day in Henry's room in the pediatric intensive care unit at University of Minnesota Children's Hospital. As Henry lay still in a room that was steadily filling with medical equipment to pump oxygen, blood, antibiotics, morphine, and nutrients into his battered, unresponsive body, just outside in the hall, Joe took his very first steps.

Every few hours, Allen updated the blog he created to update our family and hundreds of friends on Henry's condition.

Friday, December 06, 2002

Henry once again cheats death. And again it is Laurie who has to save his life—in a hospital. This morning at 7 am, Laurie called me at the Ronald McDonald house and asked that I rush to the hospital to be with her and Henry. Last night, Laurie, Jack, Joe, and I went to a Hanukah party and performance by Jack's school at a synagogue northwest of the city. It was fun and we actually saw some people there we know. Jack was awesome and it was nice to be altogether as a family, albeit minus one. We decided to leave a little early and Laurie went to the hospital (after tucking in me, Joe, and Jack) to relieve her mom and stay overnight with Henry. Before I went to sleep Laurie had called to let me know they were taking Henry for a chest x-ray because she noticed his breathing was very labored. All night long no one could get Henry comfortable. He had an oxygen mask on but he was still in trouble. By this morning, Henry took a precipitous downturn. His blood gasses were drawn and it was obvious to the PICU doctors who were being consulted by the Peds staff that he needed to be intubated. They rushed him to the Intensive Care side of the floor. Before they could get the breathing tube into him, his pulse went faint, his heart stopped beating, and he stopped breathing. CPR was done and adrenaline was administered. They got his heart functioning again and proceeded to intubate him. He is now on a ventilator. In addition to the tube down his throat, a new central line was placed in his groin going up to his heart. Henry has been given medication to paralyze him, so his body can focus on essential life sustaining functions.

The preliminary judgment of the doctors is that Henry has an infection and when they administered antibiotics to treat that infection, toxins were released into his body. I think this is called sepsis or septic shock. There is a mass of fluid in his lung which they now are draining. He is in very critical condition. My sister flew in immediately. Laurie's sister, dad, and my best friend Bill are all in transit. Henry isn't going to die. In fact, if the infection is pneumonia and they can treat it successfully, then hopefully the pain in his shoulder will be resolved. Whenever Henry has pneumonia, his shoulder hurts him terribly.

Right now he is laying catatonic on the bed with a plastic pillow of warm air bringing up his body temperature, which is kinda low. I am holding his hand (when not typing) and I talk to him a little bit, though I know he cannot hear me. I was just telling Laurie how a day or two ago, I told Henry that my goal was for him to feel well enough for me to give him a big hug. His body's fragility has robbed us of the physical contact that I love so much. Laurie said last night he sat on her lap on the wheelchair ride to radiology and she was in heaven. We're waiting for a blood transfusion, but in a snafu the blood bank hasn't readied any. He is stable. This is sad.

Monday, December 09, 2002

Henry is laying there like one big bloated catatonic boy. We talk to him all of the time like he can hear us. It is incredibly painful to do this. We talk in that loud voice one uses when they talk long distance on a cell phone, like it's going to make any difference. Putting lotion on his body is a treat. We keep him all lubed up and moving from side to side. I hope that touch really does heal. It is sad that you cannot hold or hug him with all of the tubes and wires that have sprouted out of his body.

One thing that has been really bugging me the past 72 hours is that I cannot remember Henry from any time before 7 am on Friday morning. It is so strange not to be able to remember the past 7 years at all. I cannot bring into focus any images of Henry playing, singing, fighting with jack, swimming, eating, cuddling, reading, hitting a baseball, kicking a soccer ball, watching movies, dancing, anything. I have stayed home and taken care of him the past two years and my memory is blank. It is like how my memory of my mom is frozen on the day she died. To correct this I am going to watch a copy of the *Nightline* DVD that we brought with us. Henry was featured on it earlier this year and they captured a lot of good footage of Henry being Henry. I cannot wait. I have a feeling this will make me cry a lot. I keep having this headache (so does Laurie) that is a result of not crying but feeling like I have to cry. When you weep a lot you get a headache. I wonder what is behind that phenomenon. Why does the body punish you for crying. Everyone always says, "Go ahead and cry."

Tuesday, December 10, 2002, at 10:57 a.m.

They just dropped the bomb. The preliminary results of the bronchial lavage is aspergillus fungus. From the first days of our understanding of FA and bone marrow transplants, the doctors always cited aspergillus as the major cause of death for Fanconi transplant patients. Reported attributable mortality from invasive pulmonary aspergillosis has varied, but rates are as high as 95% in recipients of allogeneic bone-marrow transplants. They are going to get a CAT scan done and if it is localized and not spread, they will operate and remove that part of his lung. You can imagine the risks associated with this kind of major surgery. I have a sense that Laurie might want to let him go with dignity and peace and not subject him to this. This will be a most difficult conversation. Please pray or think good thoughts or whatever. I wish it wasn't this. I love my son so much.

December 10, 2002, 9:10 p.m.

Well this isn't Hollywood or Hogwarts. My tears just didn't do it. Nor did my kisses and hugs. This afternoon we spoke at length with Henry's transplant doctor, John Wagner, who told us he wasn't entirely convinced it was aspergillus. We decided (Laurie wasn't too psyched, but did it for me) to go ahead with a lung biopsy to find out for certain if it is a bacterial or fungal infection. This was scheduled for tomorrow. About 20 minutes after we finished, a BMT fellow came over to us to explain that they just received the results of another culture confirming the presence of aspergillus. That's it. No more. Aspergillus is unbeatable, Fanconi anemia wins. This stupid genetic disease that I was sure was no match for the latest medicine and the greatest love beat us to a pulp. The ultimate defeat. We are now focused on keeping Henry comfortable. We'll discuss a strategy with the PICU attending for letting Henry go gently. Family members will start arriving tomorrow.

We want to have everyone here when Henry dies.

We will have Jack and Joe front and center. Laurie and I took Jack to dinner tonight. Jack drew a picture of the family, everyone has on kippot because of Hanukah. Henry has tubes and wires and is happy because he is out of the hospital. I explained to Jack that Henry will indeed be happy to be out of the hospital and it will happen this week. I told him that Henry fought very hard not to be sick, but in the end the sickness was stronger. I told him that Henry was coming home but he was not going to live any longer. I told him that we are going to have a funeral and we need Jack to help bury Henry just like he buried Grandma. I told him that Henry loves Jack and Henry knows that Jack loves Henry. He sat in Laurie's lap with his arms around her and wept. I told him that he didn't need to be strong. Laurie explained that she was crying because she is so sad and it is just fine for Jack to cry as much as he needs.

I dropped Laurie off at the hospital and went to take a shower at the Ronald McDonald house. The water would only get lukewarm.

Laurie is writing a eulogy. She is writing a book about our life trying to save Henry's life. I started this diary to help her understand the chronology of this visit, which was supposed to be a short one, and what I have been feeling. I didn't know this would become the final chapter. As hard as it might seem to believe, I really thought Henry would be President of the United States one day. I thought he had the wisdom and disposition for the job (like his mother, but I don't think she needs the headache). I am not comfortable writing about him in the past tense. It'll take some getting used to. I don't think I'll be able to say anything at the funeral. I want to make a CD of Henry's favorite music and have it duplicated and hand it out at the ceremony. Then people can take it home and always think about this special guy every time they listen to the music. I know I'll be thinking of him every waking moment and when I sleep. I just want the good memories back. I know we rode the roller coaster at the Mall of America last month. I just can't get the picture in my head.

We've been saying good-bye for a while now, but it isn't very easy. The fact that his body is here but everything else is checked out is a good thing. It gets you used to him not being around. Jack has just come over and is going to have a sleepover at the hospital with me and Laurie. Tomorrow he has a class field trip to a nature center. He loves that stuff. He'll be okay. Joe is probably too young to know anything is wrong. Maybe he does and that is why he won't stop smiling and walking and giving us joy.

How incredibly lucky I've been to not only know Henry, but to be loved by him and to be his constant companion for so long. After two years of hanging with Henry, I guess it is time for me to go home, love Laurie, Jack and Joe, find a job, and get on with life. So long, my superhero.

Wednesday, December 11, 2002, at 8:34 a.m.

We chose what day and time Henry was born, and now we'll do the same with his death. Everyone is in. My friend, (Rabbi) David Abramson, cannot be back from Israel in time to officiate at the funeral. The path is clear.

Laurie and I have been able to grab a few minutes together here and there, and we've had great conversations about Henry. Thank God for Laurie's amazing memory. She is helping me because I am still a blank. She reminded me how when Henry learned her cell phone number he became a big abuser. He'd call it every chance he got and left messages like, "Hi mom, It's Henry. I am just calling you to tell you how happy I am, how much I love you and how beautiful you are. See ya." He'd do this over and over.

I'm glad my mom isn't alive for this. But I am sad that my dad is physically alone. We are here for him, as is my sister and his friends, but how hard it must be not to have someone to lay next to in bed and talk about how much you loved your grandson and hear that everything will be all right. Henry loves all of his grandparents, aunts, uncles, great aunts, great uncles and friends so much.

December 11 at 11:11 a.m.

I went with my dad and Jack to get Jack some big boy clothes for the funeral. I also bought Henry the biggest Swiss Army knife they make. He always wanted one, but Laurie knew he was still too young. He doesn't have much of a palm, but I put his fingers around it and he is holding it now. Also, it is pretty ironic that we took Jack to get something to wear when he couldn't care less. Henry was the real clotheshorse in the family. He had style.

The clerk at the store asked if we were out having a shopping day. I wish I had the wherewithal to say, "No, we're removing life support from my son today."

We're working on funeral and burial arrangements now. I ran into the manager of the Ronald McDonald house earlier and I found that I had to actually say, "My son is going to die today and we are going to be out of here by tomorrow morning."

December 11 at 12:27 p.m.

I am very scared that we only have a few hours left with Henry. Laurie and I both had the same thought. What do we do tonight after he dies? We aren't home. Maybe we'll drive around the lakes and as Laurie suggested eat some of Henry's favorite foods, skittles, garlic bread, chips, chocolate croissants, and other nutritionally-deficient items.

December 11 at 1:26 p.m.

Dr. Wagner was just in and we all sat around reminiscing about Henry. The one thing that struck me is that Henry always said, "Let's just get it over with," or "Let's do this already," when he was going to have a procedure, or had to get blood drawn or had to go to clinic. He was impatient for the not-so-fun stuff to be over so he could get back to the good things in life. I know that Henry is glad that we are following his instructions and "just getting this over with."

They have him on Pentobarbital which keeps him very relaxed and in a dreamlike state. We'll remove a lot of the tubes and the ventilator at 6 pm. We will get everything out of his mouth so we can kiss him. Hopefully we'll be able to cradle him in our arms. We'll play his favorite songs (my brother-in-law brought some of Henry's mixed CD's from home) and probably tell some good Henry stories. A rabbi will be with us and we'll say the Vidui prayer and the Shema. I think I'll go swipe the menorah from the lobby of the hospital and we can break the rules and light the candles. Henry's last words to Laurie were, "Mom, this is a terrible last day of Hanukah."

Maybe we can make it better.

On December 11 at 6:40 p.m. CST, Allen wrote the final posting in the blog: *Henry Strongin Goldberg died. I removed his breathing tube and his heart stopped beating while Laurie held him in her arms on a rocking chair in his room.*

*F*ive-year-old Jack, one-year-old Joe, Allen's dad and my parents, all of our siblings, my aunt, and Dr. Wagner stood by as Allen and I, with the guidance of doctors, removed Henry's chest tube, arterial line, feeding tube, breathing tube, IVs, and chest leads. The official cause of death was aspergillus, an untreatable fungal infection in Henry's lung.

But it was really the failure of preimplantation genetic diagnosis that killed my son.

I removed the picture of Henry in his Batman costume that we had posted on his hospital room doors for more than two and a half years and taped it to the shroud that covered his defeated body so the people at the morgue would know who they were dealing with. Then Henry disappeared forever.

The next night, millions learned of Henry's death directly from Ted Koppel as *Nightline* rebroadcast its show on Henry's life.

From there, things unfolded much as I had imagined they would. My brother took care of all the funeral arrangements, including transporting Henry's body from Minneapolis to Washington. My sister bought me clothes to wear to Henry's funeral. I put down on paper the eulogy I had been writing and rewriting in my head for years. With significant help from my friend Erica Antonelli, Allen created a CD of Henry's favorite songs, including "Pierre," "Homemade Lemonade," "Henry You're Our Superhero," and a selection of Dan Zanes songs, to give to everyone who came to our house to sit shiva, a Jewish ritual that involves visiting the home of the family in mourning each evening for one week following a funeral.

Like a lot of little girls, Bella kept a diary to record her thoughts, feelings, and highlights of her day. When I was eight, my diary featured romantic developments like "Jessica says that Larry likes me. I hope she's right"; sports highlights like "Christine and I won first place in the three-legged race in Field Day today" and embarrassing details like "Today we got our soccer trophies. Mine had boobs and all the boys laughed at me. Maybe I should join a girl's team." Unlike mine, Bella's diary betrayed a life painful beyond her years. On December 11, 2002, Bella wrote:

Dear Diary,

This evening they are going to unplug all the machines monitoring Henry. Friday will be his funeral. There is no school today so it is like everybody is taking a day off for Henry. I wish I could find the rings he gave me to wear. This is a hard time for everyone. I look at the pictures on the fridge of Henry and I. I picture Henry and I playing checkers and other games and doing stuff together. I remember the last time he came over and he read to Lauren and me. I just wish Henry could get better.

    Bella

The day of Henry's funeral was freezing cold and pouring rain, which was perfect. I felt confused and old and empty, kind of like I did in the nightmares I had over and over again. But worse. Everything was moving in slow motion. We sat in the front row of the sanctuary, which was filled with a thousand people ranging from family and friends to complete strangers. I sat between Allen and Jack, who busily played his Game Boy Advance, the one Henry bought him with his tooth-fairy money. I didn't even notice that Jack, Lisa, and Molly Nash were there, which was extraordinary, especially in light of the fact that Molly had just had surgery and was in a halo brace. I forgot how to breathe, and my hands and legs started to tingle and then go numb, along with the rest of me, so Allen gave me a little pill that allowed me to survive.

Andrew and Abby read my eulogy.

On October 25, 1995, Henry made me a mom and a better person. Before he could even smile or talk, Henry taught me what was important and what just didn't matter at all; and he taught me to savor each moment; to love; to laugh; and to dwell in possibility.

And together as a family we have done just that, packing more smile- and laugh-producing times together in seven years than many do in a lifetime. We have lived and loved as though we could one day lose Henry while simultaneously pushing love and science to their limit to ensure that we would have him in our lives forever. Henry has driven a tractor, fallen in love, danced with ten women at one time, and laughed until he fell over. Just two days ago, Henry finally got the biggest, baddest Swiss Army knife, which he held on to until the very end. We lived every day with Henry to its fullest. We have had ice cream for dinner, transitioned from the hospital to running a lemonade stand in a matter of minutes, gone to Cactus Cantina seven nights a week, acquired every single Pokémon figure made. At last count we had 188. He met President Clinton, Cal Ripken, Batman, the entire Minnesota Twins baseball team, and more significantly, they got to meet him. We did all those things because at that moment in time we could and because, though we always hoped things would get better, we knew enough to go when the going was good. Just in case.

As I'm sure all of you know, Henry just made everything better. He was wise well beyond his years, and he was so much fun. It's almost as if all the good things in life were created with Henry in mind. No one had greater appreciation for Disney World, Funland, Sullivan's, or any of the other fun things in life than Henry. He was a great lover of music, and could sing "Brick House" and dance with the best of them. I will cherish my memories of Allen and Henry dancing together in our home. . . .

My dad used to tell me that a day without me was a day without sunshine. Now I know what he was talking about. Sweetie, you are everything enjoyable in life. You are a lemonade stand on a hot summer day. You are the first piece in a box of Godiva chocolate; kite flying on the beach; the final encore at a Springsteen show; S'mores at a campfire; a piñata at a birthday party; fireworks on the fourth of July; a ride on a Ferris wheel; the glow of candlelight during a thunderstorm; finding a sand dollar on the beach; penny candy; class outside; the last ski run of the day; meeting your child for the first time. The loss of you drenches my heart in sorrow.

I'm not sure how Cactus Cantina or Max's Ice Cream will survive without you, and I sure wish that Daddy, Jack, Joe, and I didn't have to. I miss you so, so much already. Our job now is to ensure that everything is better because of you. So, like you, we will draw our swords, but don't expect the same resiliency. You set the bar high. Give us a while and we will make you proud, my son.

$\mathcal{M}$y eulogy was followed by others by Henry's rabbis, doctors, elementary school principal, and other family members.

After the service, we filed into a black limousine, but this time Henry wasn't there and we weren't going to Disney World. Thankfully Jack and our niece Hannah were there, otherwise the silence would have been deafening. The thud of the dirt that hundreds of people threw on Henry's little coffin threatened to make me understand that I would never see my son again. On the way from Henry's grave back to the limousine, I walked out of my shoes and the cold mud froze my bare feet, reminding me that I was alive, which was agonizing. When we got home, Jack made a spaceship out of a big, empty cardboard box and sat alone in it in our basement while hundreds of family, friends, and strangers came to provide comfort and company. For nights or weeks (I can't remember), members of our community lovingly dropped off food for us. Lacking appetites, it went uneaten, so my friend and neighbor Debbie knew to come by late in the day to pick up the food and donate it to needy people whose grief hadn't robbed them of their desire for sustenance. To this day, lasagna represents the food of death, and I don't think I will ever eat it again.

The day of Henry's funeral, Bella added another entry:

Dear Diary,

When the funeral started, they sang a song about Henry. Mom started crying. Then they shared a story about Henry, this is how they said it: Hen loved his Sunflower teacher Liane and her daughter Isabella. Last summer, Henry was invited to Bella's ballet recital. He got all dressed up and excited and was ready for two hours before he had to go. Finally, Laurie said it was time to go. Henry said, "We first have to buy her flowers." That story made me cry. He was so sweet to me. They told many stories like that too. I ♥ my boyfriend Henry. I should probably forget about those boys from school, I'm taken.

Bella

One evening the week after Henry died, my brother gave me a copy of the eulogy he had written, but not shared, at Henry's funeral.

Laurie and Allen both, to my mind and in the words of my wife, Tracey, must be the luckiest unlucky people. They're the ones who walk into a brightly lit room and make the lights flicker. They bring energy and power into the room. They have the magic "x" factor that starts the party, that gathers the proverbial moths to the flame, the magnets into the gray of iron filings. They are magnetic. Others need to be with them, not just to touch them, but also—especially—to be touched by them. It's the opposite of the Groucho Marx adage: If they'll let you join the club, you'll join it if they'll have you, period. No questions asked. Just look at the last seven years, the last seven days. Look at the crowds, the depth of love for them and their extended family. This outpouring of love and grief and support is no accident or aberration. It's no surprise, either, to those of us lucky enough to have been touched by them.

When Henry was born, I, like others, suffered multiple personal losses. My boundless, bottomless grief for Henry, for Laurie and Allen, for my parents, for my family, and later for Jack, and then Joe, and for my own children, remains, even now, perhaps especially now, immeasurable.

Most difficult to admit, however, has been my fear of an intensely personal loss. My fear that with the gain of Henry, I lost my sister. How, I wondered, could Laurie, even Laurie!, weather this storm? Who could? Could I? During the months of Tracey's pregnancy with Emma, during those few bright months when the world remained full of possibility and wonder, before the awful words "Fanconi anemia" entered our lexicon and wracked our world, I often thought, in my darkest moments of private fear, that if I was to become the father of a sick child, I might—just might—be able to survive if only Laurie were to have a sick child too. Surely, if anyone could withstand such a travesty of justice, if anyone could put the lie to the notion that life must be fair, it would be Laurie. Together, we'd both make possible the impossible.

Laurie always has been my hero, long before she was called to act in a truly heroic way, and thus long before she truly was a hero. I mistook Laurie's early ease and success for heroism. What does it mean to be a hero in the absence of adversity? Not much, after all. It's a label, a red badge of courage, that must be hard-won through adversity, through worthy trials and tribulations. Any right-minded hero would trade the label, however high the honor, for the opportunity, the chance, to erase the need that gave rise to the honor. But that same hero, knowing that such chances are not our lot, would walk the same difficult path, and make the same personal sacrifices. That's what it means to be a hero. That's what it means to be Laurie. How I wish for a return to the days when my heroes were false, for a world in which my sister would have had no cause to demonstrate, time and again, her true heroism. The world, it seems, needs its heroes. Fortunately, I suppose, we have Laurie.

My fear over the loss of my hero has proved ill-founded, misguided, and flat wrong. Blinded by self-pity, I failed to recognize my sister's heroism in the face of the worst imaginable adversity. Bogged down in the details of medical care, in the frustrations of being unable to help, of having no problems to solve, I failed to grasp the reality of the situation. On the day, as Laurie put it, that Henry made her a mother, the doctors pronounced not just a death sentence, but one of the worst magnitude: Your beautiful child will die, but we cannot tell you when or at what cost. I don't know when Laurie fixed her course, but it's never wavered: Laurie did everything possible, and tried some things that were not, to save Henry's life. Through it all, though, she remained fixed on the other, equally weighty matter: Henry was sick, to be sure, but he was never a "sick child," and Laurie was never the "mother of a sick child."

My memory of Henry is and will always be that of a boy, just a boy, who walked through life just like his mother and father. He'd walk into a room as if to say, "Here I am," and the lights would go on. The party would start. The moths would gather. Henry was magical. He had the rare ability to put the trust in one of Laurie's favorite expressions (does she remember?), "If you're skating on thin ice, you might as well dance!" Henry's ice was the thinnest imaginable, and how he did dance!

Henry was, I know, the hero to Emma that Laurie was to me at a similar age. And he was a true hero, I know, because of the way that he lived his life and faced his own adversity and trials and tribulations. His feats of strength, courage, and bravery are legion. He won converts and attracted followers everywhere he went. If his parents and his doctors tried the impossible, it was only because Henry's spirit and spunk made possible the impossible, and so required such attempts. What strength, I wonder, have others gained from Henry's story? How many have attempted feats of seeming magic, only because they heard about Henry and thought, "If he can persevere, why not I?"

When Allen and I chose to have Jack, and then Joe, we chose life. But Henry's death has left a hole in our lives where there was once a child, a hero, a sense of purpose, and a source of boundless hope. There is so much about Henry, his life, and our lives with him that is overwhelmingly beautiful, dear, and immortal. And yet there is so much that is heartbreaking and wrong. That every picture of Henry has been taken. Every word of his spoken. That I will never again hold his hand, read him a bedtime story, or kiss him good night. That he is not, after all, the boy who lived. These things, even given all the enduring love, are close to unbearable.

Henry's Favorite Things

- Sidewalk chalk
  - The ice-cream man
    - Putting fish stickers on his IV bags so they look like fish tanks
  - When Max from *Where the Wild Things Are* says, "Let the wild rumpus start!"
- Squirt-gun fights
  - Snowball fights
- Jumping into piles of leaves

19

My Turn

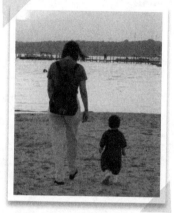

Henry walks beside me

Three weeks later, mud from the cemetery still clung to my shoes. Dressed in black, it was hard to see the torn black ribbon on my suit, or the heart still drenched in sorrow that lay within. My nine attempts to use technologically advanced genetic testing to save my boy's life and its coverage in *The New York Times Magazine* and on *Nightline* had earned me the role of "Patient Representative" at the Johns Hopkins Genetics & Public Policy Center's "Reproductive Genetics Policy: Framing the Issues" forum in Washington.

It was January 6, 2003. I sat on the dais, alongside several of the country's preeminent bioethicists and physicians, while my son Henry lay for the twenty-first day in his grave. But I tried not to think about that. Instead, I readied myself to speak for others who didn't have the opportunity to do so, to tell the seventy-five invited guests why it is so important for parents to be engaged in discussions like these, how thoughtful we are, how important this work is. I was prepared to say what I had to say and go home. I tried to convince myself that he would be there, just like he had been for seven years, six weeks, and five days.

I sat there while Dr. Mark Hughes explained the science of pre-implantation genetic diagnosis. He talked about the promise of this reproductive genetics technology to save children like Henry while ensuring that any additional children would not be born with a disease that guaranteed a short and pain-filled life. He was bright and energetic, hopeful yet realistic. His devotion to saving lives was as transparent that day as it had been when we first talked six years earlier. As I listened, I readied myself to do PGD again. After all, it was the only hope for Henry. But then I remembered why I was there: to explain what would happen if irresponsible or uninformed policymakers and bioethicists turned back the hands of time and took this science away.

As I prepared to speak, Dr. Leon Kass, a prominent bioethicist who was the head of President Bush's Council on Bioethics, was at the podium expressing fears of things that doctors are not now, and may never be, capable of doing—and things that no reasonable parent would ever do. He talked, and has written plenty, about eugenics, slippery slopes, and spare parts. He warned of a Brave New

World. At first I wondered if he was right. Were people like us hopelessly compromised when it came to making decisions on behalf of our children and children-to-be? Did we need people like him to set the rules?

As he continued to talk in abstractions, I thought about my seven-year-old son whose body was already beginning to decompose. And I thought about Molly Nash, who was back in school, playing with her friends, going to rock concerts. I thought about the promise of science, the hope that PGD offered, and the passionate commitment of doctors like Mark Hughes, Arleen Auerbach, Zev Rosenwaks, and John Wagner. I thought about the year-and-a-half delay we suffered through while politicians attempted to destroy Dr. Hughes and, ultimately, Henry's life. I thought about the fact that if such politicians had their way, then every other family with genes that cause Fanconi anemia, Tay-Sachs, sickle cell anemia, cystic fibrosis, and other devastating childhood diseases would bury their small children. I wondered if these obstructionists would change their position if their own children or grandchildren ever faced this terrifying reality. I wondered if they would sit by as they delivered babies destined to die, if they would take leave from their jobs and visit them while they underwent brain surgery, liver surgery, openheart surgery, and stem-cell transplants. I wondered if they would sit by their bedsides every day and night, watching them suffer and then fail, one organ system at a time, until they died. I wondered if they took the time to get to know any of the children and families whose futures they were threatening to destroy. Although Leon Kass never asked to, I was happy that on this day he would get to know me and my family.

Then it was my turn. I told Henry's story. I explained how we weren't looking to make Henry smarter, stronger, or more beautiful. We just wanted him to be able to be a kid and grow into a man.

PGD held the promise to make that happen. I explained that PGD isn't about creating unwanted children for their spare parts, but that it saves the new baby's life too, by showing doctors which embryos are healthy, without harm. I explained that PGD and stem-cell research aren't abstractions. They are real issues about real people. And they are the only hope for real kids like Henry. I told them what happens when PGD fails, and I introduced Sharon Harari, who told them what happens when it works.

The day after Henry died, I got a note from Sharon, which I still return to when I'm having a particularly challenging time understanding all that has happened to us. Her daughter Alma was born in January 2002, ten months before Henry died. By that time, Amitai was quite ill and needed the cord blood transplant right away. Alma was less than one month old when they did the transplant. The procedure went smoothly, and the week that Amitai went to school was the week that Henry died: "The night Henry died, I had this feeling just like I did on the millennium night. In my head I knew that after midnight our lives would continue just as they did, but my gut felt like the world might be coming to an end. If it weren't for Henry, we would have never met you. If it wasn't for you, we would have never made it through preimplantation genetic diagnosis. If it wasn't for PGD, we would have never had Alma. If it wasn't for Alma, Amitai would probably be dead today. We believe Henry saved our son's life."

And just a couple of weeks after Henry died, Allen and I received this letter:

Dear Allen and Laurie,

I don't think you know me, but boy I sure know you and Henry. I have been struggling with the right time to write this letter. I am the father of Hunter Kelley. Hunter too has Fanconi anemia. For a year and a half we searched for answers as to how to help Hunter. In 2001 we learned that PGD was now available to FAA patients. It was about this time my wife read your New York Times Magazine *article. We immediately decided we had to give PGD a try. After four cycles and many ups and downs, we got pregnant.*

On Dec. 9th, Cooper Kelley was born. A perfect match for Hunter. On January 21, Hunter underwent a transplant at University of Minnesota. Today we are back in Birmingham and Hunter is outside shooting basketball.

The reason for writing this letter is to thank you and especially thank Henry. You see, if we had never read that New York Times *article, we would have never tried PGD. Your determination to succeed at PGD gave us inspiration. Henry did not die in vain. Henry is a pioneer who has and is saving lives every day. I can only imagine what it is like to lose a son. Hopefully you can find some comfort in knowing without a doubt you and your son helped save our son's life.*

Randy Kelley

Behind every medical breakthrough are the pioneers who undergo risky, unproven treatments that fall short of their promise. It is through families like ours that doctors come to understand and perfect lifesaving treatments. Learning from our case, the doctors were able to improve the technology, and eventually science caught up with our dream. Just as research on others who came before us gave us hope for Henry, in a way we have paid our debt to them by giving others new hope.

Today, Jack is thirteen and Joe is eight. Jack has learned how to do all the things we didn't have time for while we were moving from one hospital to another, like how to swim, ride a bike, and play baseball. Two years after Henry died, as a member of the Northwest Washington Little League Orioles team, Jack hit his first grand slam. As he lay under a pile of Little Leaguers, tears were running down my cheeks. At that moment, I knew that despite everything, he was going to be OK. Among Jack's closest friends are Henry's buddies Jake, Simon, and Ari. Every year, Jack and Ari arrange a superhero toy drive in memory of Henry.

When we deliver the toys to Georgetown for the patients and their siblings, Jack reminds me that he is a sibling too, and he takes one for himself.

Joe doesn't remember much of Henry, but he reminds me a lot of him. Like Henry, Joe shares a desire to be a professional baseball player. His out-of-the-park hits and the frequency with which he runs right out of his cleats have earned him the nickname Shoeless Joe. When Joe was three, nearly every evening as we lay in bed, he would ask if Henry could come over to our house and play. When I reminded him that Henry couldn't do that because he died, Joe would ask who Henry's mother and father were. It is hard for him to understand. Me too. Now Joe has decided that Henry is with Hank Greenberg, Babe Ruth, and Lou Gehrig. All things considered, that doesn't sound so bad.

Allen started writing letters to Henry, which he posts on a blog, within days of Henry's death. For the first couple of years, Allen wrote nearly every day to let Henry know what we were up to or to tell him something interesting, or to remind him how much we all miss and love him. Here are some excerpts:

Tuesday, January 7, 2003

Dear Henry:

Another person at the conference Mommy went to was a rabbi. His name is Gerald Wolpe. He told me that he said a mishaberach for you when you were sick. He heard about you when we did the bone marrow donor drives a few years ago. His son is a Rabbi too. His name is David Wolpe and he writes books. As it happens, Mom bought me one of his books called *Making Loss Matter*. It is really interesting and helpful. Here is something he wrote:

"The times when we feel utterly defeated are the moments when we have the chance to see farther, to reach down deeper into ourselves, to acquire wisdom. It is the time to begin dreaming wise dreams."

In another part of the book, he writes: "Superheroes of children's comic books are projections of the child's imagining the power to change the world."

What that means, I think, is that you became Batman so that you could use your superpowers to make you not sick. It worked. When you were Batman, you weren't sick. Mommy bought me a little Swiss Army knife, much smaller than your humongous one, that she had engraved to say, "Batman Forever." It means a lot to me. I took your Swiss Army knife to this place that engraves things and I had them write on it "Jack—With Love, Henry." I will give it to him, from you, when he turns 9 or 10 years old.

One thing that I was thinking about the other day is how incredibly brave you always were when you went to have surgery. It was nothing to you, like you were being led away to get a haircut or something. But most kids and a lot of adults get really scared when they have to have surgery. And just because you did it so much didn't mean that you had to be brave or act like it was no big deal. You would say goodbye to me and Mom just like you did when we took you to school the first day. There were no tears, no looking back. You never knew how brave you were. I did. Mom did.

At the conference we said goodbye to Sharon, Mark, Arleen, and Zev. It was good to see them. Suzanne is going to come over soon to say hello. We gave her the blood pressure machine and we want to give her the new jog stroller for one of the kids at the clinic. I am sorry you never got to wheel around in that thing.

I have to send your death certificate to Northwest Airlines to get a refund for the tickets you and I didn't use. I remember the flight to Minnesota. You slept next to me stretched out across the seats. We sat in the back to be away from people. I was afraid someone would get you sick. You didn't want to wear your mask because it was uncomfortable, so I said okay. I bought you all of those Star Wars activities books right before we left. You liked doing the word find puzzles. Do you remember the ones that I made for you on the computer with the names of all of your cousins hidden in it? That was fun. You were really good at that and hospital bingo. I am sorry I didn't let you call in to tell your joke. The honest truth was that I didn't understand it. But it made you laugh and that made me laugh and I should have had you call it in. Oh well.

I am a little sleepy now and I think I'll curl up and take a nap. We have your bears, the mommy and baby ones that we bought at Pottery Barn Kids, and your blanket and your Henry pillow on our bed. Mom and I each grab something to hold on to when we go to bed. I think I'll hold the mommy bear. You know I wish I was holding you.

I love you.

Dad

p.s. I just thought of two things that we found so funny over the years. You did a great job doing different voices—and you were never grumpy or boring.

"You must be grumpy."
Snow White to Grumpy

"Spongebob, can you keep it down, I'm trying to be boring."
Spongebob, imitating Squidward

October 3, 2006

Dear Henry,

Okay, the weirdest thing happened on Yom Kippur. I dropped everyone off at Adas [our synagogue] and then parked down Porter Street right on the edge of Rock Creek Park. When we were walking back down the street after services, I explained to Jack that I really like that we go to synagogue in the city.

One of my favorite things to do for the High Holidays is to crush acorns. Shoes with a hard heel (which I never really wear the rest of the year) are my weapon of choice for all of the acorns that fall out of oak trees that line the streets here in DC. I love stomping those suckers.

When we got to the car, I opened up the door and Jack said there was a bird in the car. I looked and sure enough there was a little bird with a yellow belly and grey feathers on his wings. I opened the other door and the sun roof so he'd fly out. Instead of flying out, he flew from the back of the car straight into the inside of the windshield. He then positioned himself on the dashboard and closed his eyes. Everyone thought he was sleeping. It was way too fast for me. I thought that he was pretending to be asleep so we'd leave him alone.

I asked Jack what kind of bird he was and of course Jack told me exactly what kind of bird he was. A finch. I had no clue. Thank god for Jack.

I took an umbrella we had in the car and tried to nudge the finch out. He opened his eyes but had no interest in taking off. I softly prodded him a bit more but he wasn't budging. Finally, I snaked the umbrella under him and he had no choice but to stand on the umbrella. I brought him out of the car and he just stood there on the umbrella with no intention of flying away. I brought him close so everyone could check him out. He was really beautiful. There was no sign that he was hurt or that his wings were injured.

I gently stroked his feathers. Joe not-so-gently poked him. He stayed put.

I said that I was sure the bird was you. Mom said that was doubtful 'cause she is sure you are a praying mantis. I wanted to take him home since he didn't seem to want to be away from us. No one thought that was a good idea. I always think that when we have an interesting or close call with nature, you are somehow involved.

Finally I placed him up on a stone wall away from the road. He stood there for a second and then flew up into a tree. It was the strangest thing.

I was listening to the radio tonight and heard an interview with John Lennon's son, Sean. John was in the Beatles. You liked them. Sean said that he got into his car one day and when he turned the key, the radio blared out, "Darling Sean." Those are the last two words of the song that his dad recorded called, "Beautiful Boy." His dad was killed in New York when Sean was young.

Sean said that he was having a bad day and when he heard those words from his father on the radio he was comforted. He said he didn't totally understand how the universe works, but it was a nice moment. That is how I felt about the bird.

Love,

Dad

$\mathcal{I}$ didn't know what to do or where to go without Henry in my life. For seven years, our mobile party traveled wherever Henry's health determined we needed to be. His inspiring attitude paired with his serious illness gave me something to fight hard for every day. The moment-to-moment lack of urgency that followed Henry's death left me rudderless. Even more difficult, it gave me time to absorb the overwhelming feeling of utter failure that didn't have time to haunt me while Henry was alive. Clinging to the edge of a black hole that threatened to steal me away, I held true to the commitment I made, and reaffirmed, when I got pregnant with Jack and then Joe: I would not only survive, I would give my boys a great and full life, enriched by their older brother and the knowledge that Allen and I didn't just say we would do anything for our children, we had proved it.

Just as at the beginning of Henry's illness, I knew I could move forward as long as I had something I could do. I continued providing information, insights, and support to other families, and pushing for federal support for embryo and stem-cell research. To honor Henry's legacy of living well and laughing hard even in the face of serious illness, on October 25, 2003, on what would have been Henry's eighth birthday, Allen and I established Hope for Henry Foundation. Recognizing the restorative effects of laughter and learning, and how much smiles and hope can add to a patient's quality of life and determination to get better, Hope for Henry does for other ill children what we did for Henry—fills all the time the kids are waiting to get better with fun and entertainment. We give iPods, portable DVD players, digital cameras, satellite radios, and portable game players to kids undergoing bone-marrow transplants and chemotherapy. We fill the hospital clinics with new computers so kids can IM their friends, surf the Web and play games; DVD players and movies to provide distractions; and new pianos and piano lessons so they can enjoy the benefits and pleasure of music. In 2005, in the midst of Harry Potter mania, Hope for Henry threw parties in hospitals around the country to celebrate the release of *Harry Potter and the Half-Blood Prince.* Since hospitalized kids couldn't get to the bookstore, we brought the book; chocolate frogs, capes, and wands; trivia contests; and cakes depicting Harry playing Quidditch to the hospital. The success of this party led to annual superhero celebrations, summer carnivals, Halloween parties, birthday celebrations, and more. This work has generated news coverage on ABC and CNN, in *The Washington Post* and *The Wall Street Journal,* and, more important, smiles on the faces of a lot of kids like Henry, Jack, and Joe.

Our family finally has the normalcy we were fighting so hard for. We can make plans for playdates, birthday parties, or dinners with friends with near certainty that we can see them through. I can leave work with a "to-do" list, knowing that in all likelihood I'll be back the next morning. I can buy a week's worth of groceries without it being a gamble. Our family has all the simple things we fought so hard to have with Henry. But he's not here.

Fairly late into motherhood, on parents' days at school, I peer into the lunch boxes of Jack's and Joe's friends to see what normal moms pack; and I try to relate to my friends' anxieties over the school curriculum and summer camp and other wonderfully normal concerns of lucky people like us. I work hard to balance being the proud and thankful mother of two beautiful, thriving, wonderful boys with the agony of living without Henry.

.   .   .

R ecently we took our annual trip to Funland. This time, Joe was ready to go on the Paratrooper. I handed the ride operator eight tickets, we wiggled out of our shoes, and we climbed into the sparkly gold car. As the ride got going faster and faster, Joe gave me a sideways glance and squeezed my hand. His terror and delight intermingled with laughter and screams. Each time we reached the peak of the ride we screamed and waved to Allen and Jack down below. Tears of joy and loss spilled down my face but were quickly dried by the warm summer breeze before Joe could notice them. After a family Skee-Ball tournament, a few rides on the bumper cars, and victories in the horse race and beach-ball toss, with hands filled with stuffed animals and leftover tickets, the four of us walked along the boardwalk in search of cotton candy and soft ice cream. I felt something I hadn't felt in a long time . . . happy. Henry was all around me. His laughter echoed in the waves as they playfully crashed on the shore. His spirit danced with the kites in the warm summer breeze. His smile lived on in the faces of his two beautiful brothers.

I knew then that he would be with me forever, reminding me to eat dessert first.

Epilogue

*M*ax Henry Winaker was born on a Saturday morning in July 2007. His father, Jeremy, explained, "We've been waiting for a boy. We wanted you to know as we honor your Henry's gift to us and the world."

When I first met Dr. Ali Mendelson, Max's mother, she was sitting in the lotus position on the edge of Henry's bed at Georgetown. The lights were off, their eyes were closed, arms resting on their thighs outstretched, thumbs pressed to middle fingers. The only sounds were the rhythmic beating of Henry's IV pump and the soft repetitive chanting *"om"* between long deep breaths. I arrived breathless with arms filled with containers of Pringles from the basement vending machine. By that point the chemo had pretty much limited Henry's taste buds to salty food, so I acquired enough to last the day. I quietly put the stash on his bed tray next to his Pokémon figures, which waited mid-battle. I listened to the mesmerizing sound and took a deep breath, something that felt like a luxury amid the chaos of our life.

Ali Mendelson is a smart, straight talker, meticulous in her patient care. She, like so many before her, had fallen for Henry. More than one of Henry's doctors explained to me that to endure as a pediatric hematologist/oncologist—a doctor searching for cures for as-yet incurable diseases—you have to create an emotional divide between yourself and your patients and their families. Objectivity requires detachment from the heightened emotions of the moment. It also potentially offers these doctors needed breathing room to focus on the big picture—new treatments and new cures—that help current and future patients far more than providing yet another shoulder to cry on. Because this line of work nearly guarantees early and frequent exposure to children who suffer so much and die so young, feelings of failure can overwhelm and lead to despair or a retreat to the laboratory.

Perhaps the barrier is a desperate attempt to avoid inevitable and crushing feelings of grief surrounding the reality that their idea, their protocol, failed, and the cost of that failure—a human life—was too great. But then every once in a while a kid like Henry would come along and well—forget it.

I don't know if it was when Henry whipped out his sword, stuck it in the air, looked his doctor in the eye, and said, "Bring it on" in the face of yet another IV. Or when Henry showed up for his transplant workup in his Batman costume. Or it could have been the beauty of Henry's constant smile and infectious laugh. But Henry crashed through that divide from Johns Hopkins, where his doctor confessed to putting Henry's picture on her fridge for inspiration as she fought her own illness, to Detroit, where the Wayne State University researchers were motivated by Henry's photograph while they conducted our genetic testing, to Georgetown, where he sat meditating with Dr. Mendelson. Henry's world was one filled with sunshine, laughter, and fun, and it was energizing to be part of it, perhaps especially for the doctors working so hard to beat the odds and save his life.

Over the next two months, Ali and Henry talked a lot, watched cartoons in his room, and became friends. When Henry left for that last trip to Minnesota in November 2002, he didn't get a chance to say good-bye to her.

Ali was among the dozens of doctors, nurses, social workers, and art therapists who left Georgetown the morning of December 13, 2002, to attend Henry's funeral. I didn't see her there, just like I didn't see Molly Nash and her family. As it happened, Ali sat next to someone who neither we nor Henry knew. Jeremy Winaker was the new youth rabbi at Adas Israel, our synagogue in downtown Washington, DC. Ali didn't know him either, and her innocent question of "How did you know Henry?" may have been to distract her from the painful reality that one of her young patients was dead. It being early in her career, this was likely to be one of many. When Jeremy answered that he was the new rabbi and he had heard so much about Henry that he was determined to get to know him as best as he could, even in death, Ali made the connection that her sister, also a rabbi, knew Jeremy, and had mentioned to Ali that they should meet.

One year later, Ali and Jeremy got engaged. When we received the wedding invitation in the mail, I wanted to go, but Allen thought we should do the gracious thing and decline as we were clearly "B list." That week, when the *New York Times* "Vows" reporter called to interview us for her piece on Ali and Jeremy's wedding, it was clear that Allen was mistaken. On November 13, 2004, Allen and I danced at their wedding, the first time we'd danced since Henry's death two years earlier.

I didn't have to think hard about what would be an appropriate gift to honor the birth of Henry's namesake. I sent him Batman costumes in size infant, toddler, extra-small, small, and medium. Just enough to get him started.